Spinal Surgery Biomechanics: Principles for Residents and Students

Edited by

Javier Melchor Duart Clemente

Neurosurgery and Spinal Surgery Departments
Valencia General Hospital
Valencia, Spain

Spinal Surgery Biomechanics: Principles for Residents and Students

Editor: Javier Melchor Duart Clemente

ISBN (Online): 978-981-5322-73-6

ISBN (Print): 978-981-5322-74-3

ISBN (Paperback): 978-981-5322-75-0

© 2025, Bentham Books imprint.

Published by Bentham Science Publishers Pte. Ltd. Singapore. All Rights Reserved.

First published in 2025.

need for a court order if at any point you breach any terms of this License Agreement. In no event will any delay or failure by Bentham Science Publishers in enforcing your compliance with this License Agreement constitute a waiver of any of its rights.

3. You acknowledge that you have read this License Agreement, and agree to be bound by its terms and conditions. To the extent that any other terms and conditions presented on any website of Bentham Science Publishers conflict with, or are inconsistent with, the terms and conditions set out in this License Agreement, you acknowledge that the terms and conditions set out in this License Agreement shall prevail.

Bentham Science Publishers Pte. Ltd.
80 Robinson Road #02-00
Singapore 068898
Singapore
Email: subscriptions@benthamscience.net

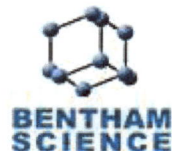

BENTHAM SCIENCE

CONTENTS

FOREWORD

When I was challenged to write an introduction to this book, I did not hesitate in accepting it, since for me as a biomedical engineer who is an expert in the field of spinal biomechanics, it has always been a passion more than a job. For the last 30 years, I have studied the biomechanics of the spine and, based on that knowledge, developed new implants and spinal prostheses that respond to clinical problems that my medical colleagues have "suffered."

But I have not only found the passion in myself; the love of the authors for the spine and for the patients behind it and to whom we all owe ourselves, is evident in all the chapters of this book. I believe that in the vast world of medicine and biomedical engineering, few fields arouse as much interest and challenge as the biomechanics of the spine, which is why I believe that the existence of this type of publication is essential. As advances occur in the study of the biomechanics of the spine, a series of crucial questions arise to be addressed that are rigorously treated in this book, from the methods to evaluate the anchorage of pedicle screws to the different techniques of total lumbar disc replacement. In summary, the chapters of the book summarized below explore in detail the scientific and medical advances that have shaped this constantly evolving area of research.

The first chapter, "Biomechanical Testing of Pedicle Screw Anchorage", looks into the testing techniques that allow a rigorous evaluation of the anchorage capacity of pedicle screws. These components are essential for the stability of the spine and their understanding is essential for successful surgical procedures. This first chapter demonstrates how science and engineering come together in the search for surgical excellence.

In chapter two, the doors open to an in-depth debate on whether total lumbar disc replacement is an option that should continue to be worked on to achieve a disc prosthesis that truly maintains the biomechanics of the spine. In a world where surgical options are increasingly varied, the chapter explores the different types of available prostheses and immerses us in the biomechanical and clinical aspects that determine when this technique should be used and in what type of patients.

In contrast to the previous chapter in the third chapter, the focus is on the study of the different techniques to achieve intervertebral fusion with an interbody cage. Here, biomechanical and biological issues such as osseointegration or the movements of adjacent vertebrae are intertwined as we delve into the study of the different techniques that have been used to create an optimal environment for bone growth between the vertebrae using the concept of inter somatic cage.

Continuing with the fourth chapter, "Management of Degenerative Spinal Conditions with Osteoporosis", what an osteoporotic vertebra is and the biomechanical behavior of an osteoporotic spine are analyzed. The above is essential to be able to understand which technique or set of surgical techniques are the most appropriate to restore the height and function of a fractured vertebra due to osteoporosis. The final part of the chapter explores the use of pedicle screws with cement, analyzing their advantages and possible complications that may appear when using these implants.

In the fifth chapter, we deal with the biomechanical causes that trigger spondylolisthesis, how they are classified, and finally how the body tries to mechanically compensate for this pathology. Finally, instructions are given on its treatment.

With chapters six and seven, our horizons on spinal biomechanics expand even further. In section six, interspinous devices are analyzed as an alternative for stabilization without fusion, making a classification of them and the consequences of their use on the biomechanics of the spine.

In the last chapter, the book immerses us in the definition of instability and in the different methodologies used throughout history to measure spinal instability, revealing how biomechanics is essential to understanding and classifying spinal injuries.

In summary, this book provides a detailed analysis of the complex biomechanical mechanisms that govern the human spine. From the evaluation of pedicle screw anchorage to innovative solutions for spinal stability, this book offers a comprehensive perspective that combines scientific research with clinical applications. Ultimately, it is a valuable source of knowledge for medical professionals, biomedical engineers, and students who wish to dig into the challenging field of spinal biomechanics and how different types of implants designed for the spine interact and restore function.

Carlos Atienza
Healthcare Technology Area
Instituto de Biomecánica de Valencia (IBV)
Valencian Community
Valencia, Spain

PREFACE

Dear colleagues, we hope you enjoy this book you have now in your hands. It started spontaneously as a group of friends of spinal surgeons thought it would be useful for the coming generations to share and put at hand this useful knowledge based on our practical experience throughout the years to improve the clinical results of spinal surgery patients.

The spine is a complex structure both from the static or anatomic point of view, as it is composed of bone (vertebrae), intervertebral discs, muscles, and ligaments (that could be the reason why the less aggressive you are, the better the outcome. It is in this complex point of intersection of statism and dynamicity where biomechanics play an important role, helping us to understand both how the spine behaves in its intact fashion and more importantly after we apply surgical gestures either for decompression or stabilization.

Biomechanics is the study of mechanics of life, and in our case, the mechanics of the moving spine. Its knowledge is key to avoiding complications during and after spinal surgery and improving clinical results by striving to get enough bony fusion and achieving good sagittal balance. As important as which patient should be operated on and when, the answers of why and how are also important to achieve success. That is why it is so important to know and understand the basic concepts with the intent to try to best help our patients who need spinal surgery.

This book does not pretend to be extensive, but rather a start for our younger colleagues. It is focused on the lumbar spine, starting with a chapter on biomechanical testing of the pedicle screw, which is the cornerstone of instrumented lumbar fusion. Before dealing with different fusion techniques in the third chapter, the second chapter deals with the motion-sparing technique of disc replacement. Fixation in osteoporotic patients and interspinous stabilizers have also been discussed, playing a role in lumbar surgery. Finally, the last chapter deals with the biomechanical view of fracture classifications. We hope you enjoy it and find these few chapters useful. This content of the book will surely help in the care of spine health.

Javier Melchor Duart Clemente
Neurosurgery and Spinal Surgery Departments
Valencia General Hospital
Valencia, Spain

List of Contributors

Anna Spicher	Department of Orthopaedics and Traumatology, Medical University of Innsbruck, Innsbruck, Austria
Amparo Vanaclocha	Biomechanical Institute of Valencia, Valencia, Spain
Asad Lak	University of Iowa Hospitals and Clinics, Department of Neurosurgery, Iowa City, Iowa, Unites States
Clayton Rosinski	University of Iowa Hospitals and Clinics, Department of Neurosurgery, Iowa City, Iowa, Unites States
Eva Díez-Sanchidrián	Faculty of Medicine, University of Santiago de Compostela, Santiago de Compostela, Spain
Enrique Marescot-Rodríguez	Orthopedics Department, Pontevedra University Hospital, Pontevedra, Spain
Eva Díez-Sanchidrián	Faculty of Medicine, Santiago de Compostela University, Santiago, Spain
Félix Tomé-Bermejo	Spinal Unit, FJD, Madrid, Spain
Javier Melchor Duart Clemente	Neurosurgery and Spinal Surgery Departments, Valencia General Hospital, Valencia, Spain
Javier Cuarental García	Spinal Unit, FJD, Madrid, Spain
Javier Melchor Duart-Clemente	Neurosurgery and Spinal Surgery Departments, Valencia General Hospital, Valencia, Spain
Javier Melchor Duart-Clemente	Neurosurgery and Spinal Surgery Departments, Valencia General Hospital, Valencia, Spain
Luis Álvarez-Galovich	Spinal Unit, FJD, Madrid, Spain
Luis Puente-Sánchez	Spinal Unit, Orthopedics Department, University Hospital Complex of Santiago de Compostela, Santiago de Compostela, Spain
Luis Álvarez-Galovich	Spinal Unit, FJD, Madrid, Spain
Máximo Alberto Díez-Ulloa	Spinal Unit, Orthopedics Department, University Hospital Complex of Santiago de Compostela, Santiago de Compostela, Spain
Máximo-Alberto Díez-Ulloa	Spinal Unit, Orthopedics Department, University Hospital Complex of Santiago de Compostela, Santiago, Spain
Mani Sandhu	University of Iowa Hospitals and Clinics, Department of Neurosurgery, Iowa City, Iowa, Unites States
Nieves Saiz-Sapena	Consortium General University Hospital of Valencia, Valencia, Spain
Pablo Jordá-Gómez	General University Hospital of Castellon, Valencia, Spain
Parchi Paolo Domenico	1st Orthopedic and Traumatology Division, Department of translational research and new technology in medicine and surgery, University of Pisa, Pisa, Italy
Patrick W. Hitchon	University of Iowa Hospitals and Clinics, Department of Neurosurgery, Iowa City, Iowa, Unites States

Richard Lindtner   Department of Orthopaedics and Traumatology, Medical University of Innsbruck, Innsbruck, Austria

Vicente Vanaclocha   University of Valencia, Faculty of Medicine, Av. de Blasco Ibáñez, 15, 46010 Valencia, Spain

Werner Schmoelz   Department of Orthopaedics and Traumatology, Medical University of Innsbruck, Innsbruck, Austria

CHAPTER 1

Biomechanical Testing of Pedicle Screw Anchorage

Werner Schmoelz[1,*], **Richard Lindtner**[1], **Anna Spicher**[1], **Luis Álvarez-Galovich**[2] and **Javier Melchor Duart Clemente**[3]

[1] *Department of Orthopaedics and Traumatology, Medical University of Innsbruck, Innsbruck, Austria*

[2] *Spinal Unit, FJD, Madrid, Spain*

[3] *Neurosurgery and Spinal Surgery Departments, Valencia General Hospital, Valencia, Spain*

Abstract: This chapter provides an overview of biomechanical *in vitro* testing of pedicle screws. Several aspects, such as specimen selection, test setup, and loading modalities for the investigation of screw anchorage are discussed. In general, cement augmentation is an effective technique to improve pedicle screw anchorage. However, in clinical practice, it should be considered that augmentation is most effective in the osteoporotic bone while in healthy bone, the improvement of screw anchorage is only marginal.

Keywords: Augmentation, Loading protocol, PMMA cement, Pedicle screws, Screw loosening, Screw failure.

INTRODUCTION

In the last decades, the use of pedicle screws has become standard for dorsal instrumentations in modern spine surgery for many pathologies. Different conditions in morphology and bone quality in degenerative, deformity, trauma and tumor surgery have led to adaptions and modifications of the traditional pedicle screw concept. To enhance pedicle screw anchorage and reduce the risk of loosening, augmentation techniques with PMMA cement and alternative materials were developed and established in clinical practice. Other options to increase pedicle screw anchorage without increasing the overall rigidity of the instrumentation are modifications in the screw design, such as adaption of the thread, screw core diameter, expandable screws, or osteointegrative coatings of the screws [1-5].

---

* **Corresponding author Werner Schmoelz:** Department of Orthopaedics and Traumatology, Medical University of Innsbruck, Innsbruck, Austria; E-mail: werner.schmoelz@i-med.ac.at

In scoliotic deformities or hyperkyphotic spines, the research focus often shifts from the improvement of screw anchorage to the possibility of applying forces and moments with implanted pedicle screws to perform derotation, compression, and tension maneuvers to selected vertebrae, in order to correct the deformity. For this purpose, modified and long screw heads with reposition possibilities were developed.

In the implementation of design modifications and the development of novel pedicle screw designs, *in vitro* biomechanical investigation with cadaver specimens plays an important role in anticipating the effect and functionality of the implants and their later clinical performance. Therefore, *in vitro* biomechanical experiments are an important link between the development and clinical application of novel implants and surgical techniques.

The obvious advantages of biomechanical investigations prior to clinical trials are their relatively easy feasibility and the possibility of a direct comparison with current standard techniques using standardized protocols in a controlled lab environment with limited confounding factors. However, the clinical relevance of biomechanical *in vitro* investigations can vary with the experimental design and execution.

In the following lines, biomechanical testing methods for the evaluation of pedicle screw anchorage are briefly described and discussed. Additionally, selected studies investigating pedicle screw anchorage of various screw designs and augmentation techniques are presented, too.

MATERIALS

Specimens

Bone quality and donor characteristics such as age, sex, bone mineral density (osteoporotic, osteopenic or normal), and grade/state of degeneration can vary widely and may have a significant effect on the results. Therefore, selected specimens must be appropriate and suitable for the postulated hypothesis and study aim. Specimens of various origins as well as artificial bone surrogates or human cadaver tissue can be utilized for biomechanical testing. Due to the limited availability and legal handling requirements of human vertebral bodies, biomechanical testing is also conducted with ovine, bovine or porcine vertebral bodies. However, differences in the bone properties, anatomy, and morphology of animal specimens should be considered in the interpretation of the results and the transfer of the results to clinical practice [6].

With the use of human specimens, ethical considerations and specimen handling must be clarified and settled with the local ethical institutional review board prior to the start of testing [7]. Another relevant point to be considered with the use of human specimens is specimen preservation. It must be distinguished between fresh frozen and embalmed (*e.g.* Alcohol-Glycerin, formalin, Thiel fixated, *etc.*) specimens. In a study comparing the biomechanical properties of formalin-fixed and fresh frozen functional spinal units (FSU), it was reported that embalmed specimens do not resemble *in vivo* features and show significantly different biomechanical properties than fresh frozen specimens [8]. Regarding the effect of preservation methods on bone tissue, Unger *et al.* compared three preservation methods with fresh frozen bone tissue and concluded that embalming significantly alters the mechanical properties of bone tissue, and the use of embalmed specimens should be restricted to pilot tests [9]. In the literature, fresh frozen specimens are considered the gold standard. After slow thawing, they should be kept wet with saline solution during testing, and at room temperature. Also, test duration should be kept constant for reliable and reproducible results of the biomechanical experiments [10].

For clamping and fixation of the specimens in the test setup to enable mechanical loading, specimens are usually embedded in plastics (*e.g.* Poly-methyl-methacrylate (PMMA) or Epoxy -resin). The rigidity of the embedding on the tested structure as well as the stiffness of the embedding material should also be considered in the evaluation and interpretation of the measured physical parameters.

Biomechanical Testing

In the last decades, biomechanical test methods were continuously refined and adapted to implement new insights and knowledge in the engineering of material testing, *in vivo* measurements, and anatomy. This allowed a more realistic simulation of clinical conditions and to investigate relevant research questions as physiologically as feasible. In the following, two test methods to investigate pedicle screw anchorage are described.

Test Setups for Pedicle Screw Pull-Out Tests

Initial, simple, and quick experimental comparisons of varying screw designs or augmentation techniques of pedicle screws are often conducted with axial pull-out tests. They are carried out by applying an axial load with a displacement vector co-axial to the long screw axis while the vertebral body is fixed in the test setup (Fig. **1**). After the complete pullout of the pedicle screw, the force-displacement curve is analyzed and a drop in the force plot (*e.g.* 25% of maximal force) is considered a failure of the screw anchorage.

This kind of experimental biomechanical testing is relatively simple and quick. However, the clinical relevance of pull-out tests for thoracolumbar pedicle screws is questionable. In particular, in pullout tests with cadaver specimens, a very high non-physiological failure load and a failure pattern not reflecting the clinical failure mode are often reported for cement-augmented pedicle screws. These high failure loads are due to pedicle avulsion fractures occurring while the cement cloud still attached to the screw is pulled through the pedicle. Additionally, *in vivo* studies of patients with instrumented implants have shown that during everyday activities, thoracolumbar pedicle screws are mainly subjected to a cranio-caudal axial loading with a superimposed bending moment; the absolute load magnitude varies strongly depending on the patients and the indication for the instrumentation [11, 12]. A mainly axial force co-axial to the long screw axis as applied in pull-out tests was not reported in the *in vivo* studies of patients with instrumented implants.

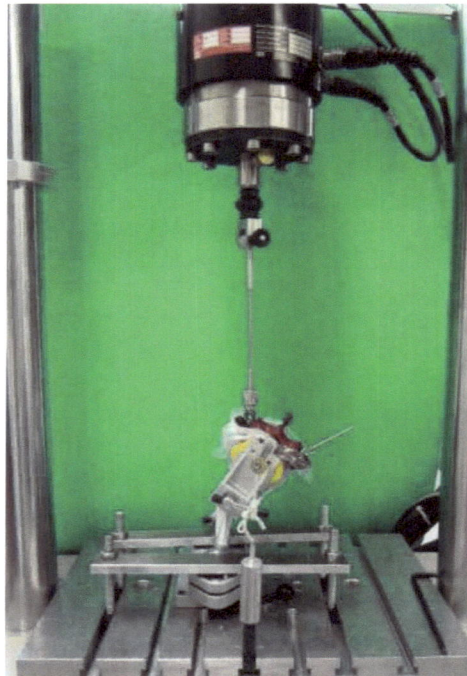

Fig. (1). Test setup of a typical pull-out test with the vertebral body embedded in PMMA and fixed in a ball joint vice to align the long axis of the screw with the displacement vector applied by a material testing machine.

Test Setups for Cyclic Craniocaudal Loading of Pedicle Screws

Principally, there are two test models for experimental *in vitro* testing of pedicle screw anchorage in anatomic specimens with cyclic cranio-caudal loading. On one hand, an experimental test setup comprising the full pedicle screw construct with functional spinal units and 4 or more pedicle screws being loaded simultaneously [13, 14]; and, on the other hand, the experimental test setup with isolated vertebrae loading each pedicle screw individually [3, 5, 15, 16]. With the former (loading of the full pedicle screw construct with multiple screws), the instrumentation can be loaded and tested comparably to its clinical routine application. Regarding the test setup, this model is closely adapted to ASTM or ISO standard tests developed for the mechanical evaluation and fatigue testing of pedicle screw constructs. However, due to their different initial purpose, an analysis of the anchorage of the full construct or the detection of a single loose pedicle screw is hardly possible. Additionally, the sample size required for a comparison of two different techniques for pedicle screw anchorage is substantially higher. This is due to interindividual differences in the bone quality and pedicle morphology of the tested vertebrae causing a wide spreading and variance in the obtained results.

In contrast to loading and testing the full construct of instrumentation, loading each pedicle screw individually allows a comparison of two screw anchorage techniques in the left and right pedicle of one vertebral body with comparable pedicle morphology and bone quality. Thereby, also smaller differences in pedicle screw anchorage of the two techniques can be detected and studied with an acceptable and still feasible sample size because the difference in bone quality and morphology of the left and right pedicle can be assumed negligible.

Various research groups developed experimental test setups and loading protocols to evaluate the anchorage of single isolated pedicle screws; they all vary to a certain extent. However, they all have in common that they use a material testing machine to apply a cyclic, predominantly craniocaudal oriented, load resulting in a combination of a craniocaudal oriented force superimposed by a bending moment in flexion (Fig. **2a**). During cyclic loading, compensatory motions (open degrees of freedom) are enabled to allow tilting and loosening of the pedicle screw inside the pedicle and vertebral body to replicate the clinical failure mode.

Loading Protocol

Cyclic loading of pedicle screws to provoke loosening can be conducted either with constant force limits (*e.g.* between 50 and 200N) or with stepwise or continuously increasing force limits. An increasing load amplitude is often used for comparisons of screw anchorage in varying bone quality or for comparison of augmented and non-augmented pedicle screws. It is well suited to provoke loosening/failure of screw anchorage in anatomical specimens with expected variations in screw anchorage properties. Cyclic loading can be applied either in force control with a set loading frequency or in displacement control with force limits. While the latter keeps the loading rate constant, a set loading frequency causes an increase in the loading rate with higher loads and increasing elastic deformation.

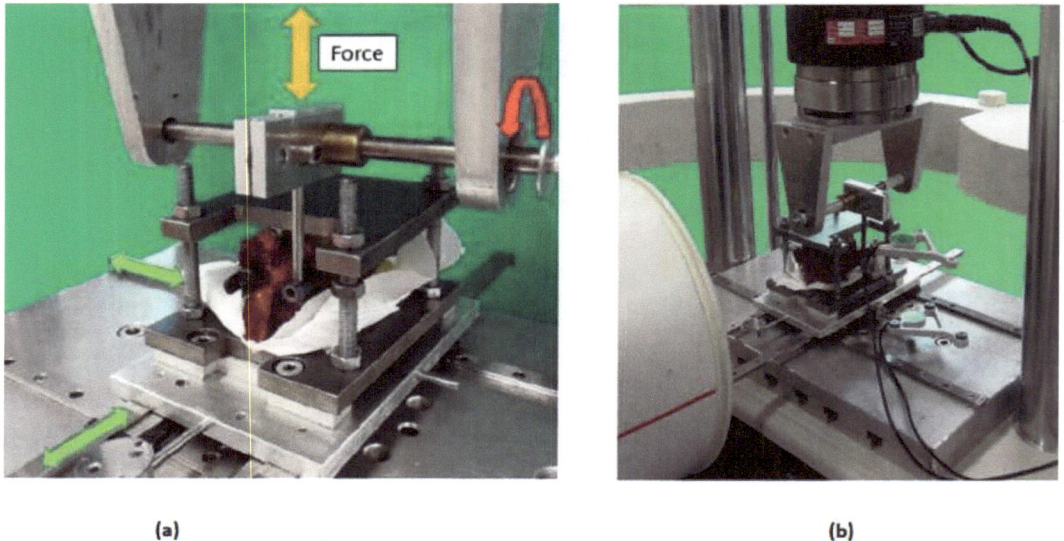

(a) (b)

Fig. (2). (**a**) Exemplary test setup for cyclic craniocaudal loading of a pedicle screw: translational degrees of freedom in green, rotational degrees of freedom in red and force application in yellow, (**b**) 3D motion analysis system to measure screw motion and fluoroscopy to visualize screw loosening during cyclic loading.

Evaluation of Screw Loosening

A simple, albeit relatively undifferentiated method to evaluate the loosening of a pedicle screw is a displacement limit of the actuator of the material testing machine connected to the pedicle screw head. The loosening of a pedicle screw and its motion during cyclic loading can be visualized on X-rays by placing fluoroscopy around the material testing machine during cyclic loading. With a 3D-motion analysis system fixed at the screw head, the relative motion of a pedicle screw inside a vertebral body can be quantified and used for the evaluation of screw anchorage (Fig. **2b**). For a detailed analysis and evaluation of pedicle screw anchorage in the vertebral body, the slope of the force plot during cyclic loading can be of assistance, too.

RESULTS

In the literature, there are numerous studies investigating specific research questions related to pedicle screw loosening in biomechanical *in vitro* experiments with cyclic cranio-caudal loading. A summary of three studies of our research group [1, 3, 16] -all of them using osteoporotic vertebral bodies with cement-augmented and non-augmented control pedicle screws (n=120)- shows a significant higher load at failure and significantly higher number of load cycles for cement augmented pedicle screws (Fig. **3**). It should be noted that all non-augmented control screws reached a failure load of approximately 230N, independent of screw design, screw manufacturer or the screw material. By comparison with *in vivo* forces measured in patients with instrumented implants during everyday activities [11, 12], these results and force magnitudes can be put into clinical context. With *in vivo* load magnitudes in the same range as the reported failure loads of *in vitro* experiments for non-augmented pedicle screws in osteoporotic vertebral bodies, it is well possible that pedicle screws in osteoporotic patients can loosen during everyday activities. With a cement augmentation, the load level at loosening (approximately 425N) could be elevated and was well above the range magnitude reported for patients with instrumented implants during everyday activities [11, 12].

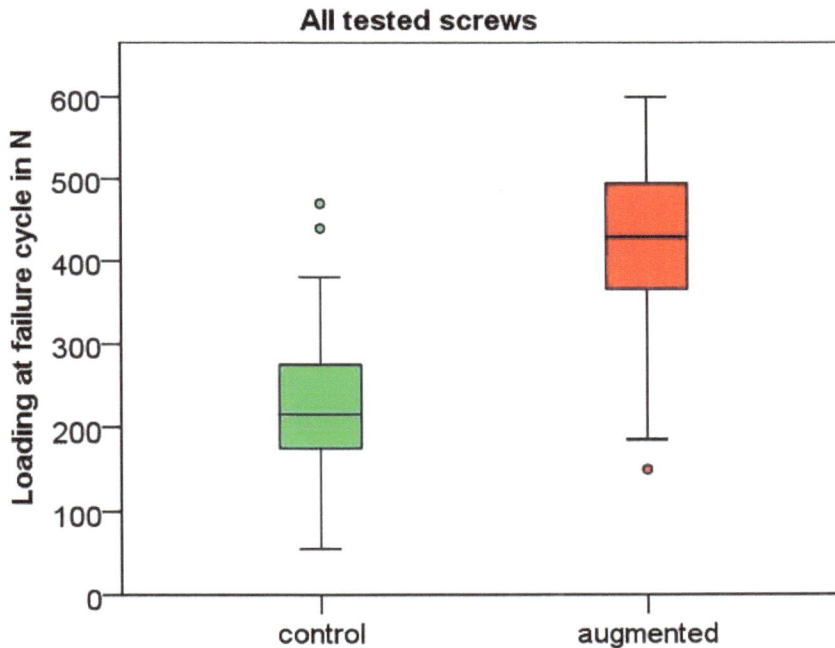

Fig. (3). Box-plot showing median and quartiles of the load level at loosening for non-augmented control and cement-augmented pedicle screws.

The studies further showed that -in osteoporotic vertebrae- the cement augmentation technique has a negligible effect on the load level at loosening. Compared augmentation techniques included *in situ* augmentation and two techniques with screw placement in the doughy not fully cured cement [1].

Varying material properties of the pedicle screws (titan alloys or carbon-fiber reinforced CF/PEEK) had no effect on the screw anchorage and the load magnitude at loosening and the positive effect of cement augmentation already shown for metallic screws could also be confirmed for non-metallic CF/PEEK screws [3].

In case a reposition maneuver *via* pedicle screws is planned, it is favorable for the screw anchorage to carry out the reposition prior to the augmentation. With this order, the maximum possible force applied during the repositioning might be limited. However, pedicle screws with compromised anchorage during the reposition can be well anchored again by *in situ* cement augmentation after the reposition [17].

With a similar test setup and craniocaudal loading of pedicle screws, Weiser *et al.* could show a significant correlation between the bone mineral density (BMD) of the vertebral body and the anchorage of pedicle screws [18]. In a further study with a wide range of the BMD in the tested vertebral bodies and a comparison of augmented and non-augmented control screws in the left and right pedicle, they reported only a significant improvement of screw anchorage by cement augmentation in osteoporotic vertebral bodies. With increasing bone mineral density, the positive effect of the augmentation on the screw anchorage decreases: while in osteopenic vertebral bodies, an effect of the augmentation could still be seen (albeit not significant), in vertebral bodies with normal BMD the cement augmentation had no effect on pedicle screw anchorage [5, 18].

Limitations of Biomechanical *In Vitro* Tests

Biological factors, such as bone healing or osteointegration of pedicle screws over time, can not be included in biomechanical *in vitro* investigations. Therefore, a statement on the clinical performance is limited to the mechanical performance of the components without consideration of biological factors. Further, compared to clinical studies the sample size of biomechanical *in vitro* investigations is smaller. However, it should be considered, that biomechanical tests are conducted in a controlled laboratory environment and often with a paired study design. Therefore, common confounding variables occurring in a clinical trial are excluded and valid conclusions are also possible with a limited sample size.

CONCLUSION

Biomechanical studies investigating pedicle screw anchorage are an important tool to the clinical arena to evaluate and further develop already available techniques, materials, and alternatives. The used test setup and loading protocol in biomechanical investigations should reflect the clinical *in vivo* conditions as physiologically as possible and feasible.

REFERENCES

[1] Bostelmann R, Keiler A, Steiger HJ, Scholz A, Cornelius JF, Schmoelz W. Effect of augmentation techniques on the failure of pedicle screws under cranio-caudal cyclic loading. Eur Spine J 2017; 26(1): 181-8.
[http://dx.doi.org/10.1007/s00586-015-3904-3] [PMID: 25813011]

[2] Frankel BM, D'Agostino S, Wang C. A biomechanical cadaveric analysis of polymethylmethacrylate-augmented pedicle screw fixation. J Neurosurg Spine 2007; 7(1): 47-53.
[http://dx.doi.org/10.3171/SPI-07/07/047] [PMID: 17633487]

[3] Lindtner RA, Schmid R, Nydegger T, Konschake M, Schmoelz W. Pedicle screw anchorage of carbon fiber-reinforced PEEK screws under cyclic loading. Eur Spine J 2018; 27(8): 1775-84.
[http://dx.doi.org/10.1007/s00586-018-5538-8] [PMID: 29497852]

[4] Viezens L, Sellenschloh K, Püschel K, *et al.* Impact of screw diameter on pedicle screw fatigue strength—A biomechanical evaluation. World Neurosurg 2021; 152: e369-76.
[http://dx.doi.org/10.1016/j.wneu.2021.05.108] [PMID: 34087457]

[5] Weiser L, Huber G, Sellenschloh K, *et al.* Time to augment?! Impact of cement augmentation on pedicle screw fixation strength depending on bone mineral density. Eur Spine J 2018; 27(8): 1964-71.
[http://dx.doi.org/10.1007/s00586-018-5660-7] [PMID: 29948322]

[6] Wilke HJ, Geppert J, Kienle A. Biomechanical *in vitro* evaluation of the complete porcine spine in comparison with data of the human spine. Eur Spine J 2011; 20(11): 1859-68.
[http://dx.doi.org/10.1007/s00586-011-1822-6] [PMID: 21674213]

[7] Riederer B, Bolt S, Brenner E, Bueno-López J, Chirculescu A, Davies DC, *et al.* The legal and ethical framework governing Body Donation in Europe – 1st update on current practice. Eur J Anat 2012; 16: 1-21.

[8] Wilke HJ, Krischak S, Claes LE. Formalin fixation strongly influences biomechanical properties of the spine. J Biomech 1996; 29(12): 1629-31.
[http://dx.doi.org/10.1016/S0021-9290(96)80016-9] [PMID: 8945663]

[9] Stefan U, Michael B, Werner S. Effects of three different preservation methods on the mechanical properties of human and bovine cortical bone. Bone 2010; 47(6): 1048-53.
[http://dx.doi.org/10.1016/j.bone.2010.08.012] [PMID: 20736094]

[10] Costi JJ, Ledet EH, O'Connell GD. Spine biomechanical testing methodologies: The controversy of consensus *vs* scientific evidence. JOR Spine 2021; 4(1): e1138.
[http://dx.doi.org/10.1002/jsp2.1138] [PMID: 33778410]

[11] Rohlmann A, Bergmann G, Graichen F. Loads on internal spinal fixators measured in different body positions. Eur Spine J 1999; 8(5): 354-9.
[http://dx.doi.org/10.1007/s005860050187] [PMID: 10552317]

[12] Rohlmann A, Graichen F, Weber U, Bergmann G. 2000 Volvo Award winner in biomechanical studies: Monitoring *in vivo* implant loads with a telemeterized internal spinal fixation device. Spine 2000; 25(23): 2981-6.
[http://dx.doi.org/10.1097/00007632-200012010-00004] [PMID: 11145808]

[13] Schulze M, Gehweiler D, Riesenbeck O, *et al.* Biomechanical characteristics of pedicle screws in osteoporotic vertebrae—comparing a new cadaver corpectomy model and pure pull-out testing. J Orthop Res 2017; 35(1): 167-74.
[http://dx.doi.org/10.1002/jor.23237] [PMID: 27003836]

[14] Spiegl UJ, Weidling M, Schleifenbaum S, Reinhardt M, Heyde CE. Comparison of long segmental

dorsal stabilization with complete *versus* restricted pedicle screw cement augmentation in unstable osteoporotic midthoracic vertebral body practures: A biomechanical study. World Neurosurg 2020; 143: e541-9.
[http://dx.doi.org/10.1016/j.wneu.2020.08.002] [PMID: 32777399]

[15]   Liebsch C, Zimmermann J, Graf N, Schilling C, Wilke HJ, Kienle A. *In vitro* validation of a novel mechanical model for testing the anchorage capacity of pedicle screws using physiological load application. J Mech Behav Biomed Mater 2018; 77: 578-85.
[http://dx.doi.org/10.1016/j.jmbbm.2017.10.030] [PMID: 29096123]

[16]   Schmoelz W, Keiler A, Konschake M, Lindtner RA, Gasbarrini A. Effect of pedicle screw augmentation with a self-curing elastomeric material under cranio-caudal cyclic loading—a cadaveric biomechanical study. J Orthop Surg Res 2018; 13(1): 251.
[http://dx.doi.org/10.1186/s13018-018-0958-z] [PMID: 30305126]

[17]   Schmoelz W, Heinrichs CH, Schmidt S, *et al.* Timing of PMMA cement application for pedicle screw augmentation affects screw anchorage. Eur Spine J 2017; 26(11): 2883-90.
[http://dx.doi.org/10.1007/s00586-017-5053-3] [PMID: 28374330]

[18]   Weiser L, Huber G, Sellenschloh K, *et al.* Insufficient stability of pedicle screws in osteoporotic vertebrae: biomechanical correlation of bone mineral density and pedicle screw fixation strength. Eur Spine J 2017; 26(11): 2891-7.
[http://dx.doi.org/10.1007/s00586-017-5091-x] [PMID: 28391382]

CHAPTER 2

Lumbar Total Disc Replacement (TDR), is it Worth it?

Vicente Vanaclocha[1,*], Amparo Vanaclocha[2], Nieves Saiz-Sapena[3], Pablo Jordá-Gómez[4] and **Javier Melchor Duart-Clemente[5]**

[1] *University of Valencia, Faculty of Medicine, Av. de Blasco Ibáñez, 15, 46010 Valencia, Spain*

[2] *Biomechanical Institute of Valencia, Valencia, Spain*

[3] *Consortium General University Hospital of Valencia, Valencia, Spain*

[4] *General University Hospital of Castellon, Valencia, Spain*

[5] *Neurosurgery and Spinal Surgery Departments, Valencia General Hospital, Valencia, Spain*

Abstract: Low back pain is a prevalent medical condition. Although most patients improve conservative treatments, some need surgery. The traditional procedure, the spinal arthrodesis, fixes a spinal segment, forcing the adjacent ones to undergo an extra load and a mobility excess that is the cause of middle and long-term discal degeneration and zygapophyseal joint arthritis changes. All this can be the source of further low back pain and require a new surgical procedure with a new spinal fusion in an average of ten years.

Joint mobility preservation is a must in all areas of surgery, and the spine is no exception. Disc arthroplasty has provided better results than spinal arthrodesis, particularly in patients under 50 with discal degeneration and no concurrent zygapophyseal joint arthritic changes. The patient selection must be accurate to get adequate results. No zygapophyseal joint damage must be present as otherwise, low back pain is common after disc arthroplasty.

The surgical technique must concentrate on every detail. The retroperitoneal approach is challenging even in the best hands. In this respect, the assistance of an access vascular surgeon is of particular help. The prosthetic disc's final position inside the discal must be no more than 2mm from the midline and 4 mm from the posterior aspect of the vertebral body. The anterior longitudinal ligament and annulus fibrosus removal induce an excess of mobility not controlled by the commercially available discal prosthesis. It is an area that still needs improvement.

The choice of which discal prosthesis to use depends on the surgeon's preferences, and new designs steadily improve the features, results, and complication rate of the previously existing ones. But there is still plenty of room for further improvement.

***** **Corresponding author Vicente Vanaclocha:** University of Valencia, Faculty of Medicine, Av. de Blasco Ibáñez, 15, 46010 Valencia, Spain; E-mail: vvanaclo@hotmail.com

Keywords: Anterior lumbar approach, Disc prosthesis, Total disc replacement.

INTRODUCTION

Chronic low back pain is frequent in the population [1 - 4] and a highly prevalent cause of temporary sick leave [5 - 7] and permanent disability [8 - 10]. Its causes include all spine components, supporting structures, ligaments, and muscles [11 - 13].

A significant percentage of these patients are young people [14] under 50 years of age [15], in whom this type of pain causes substantial negative consequences for their quality of life [16] and work opportunities [17 - 19].

Although degenerative disc disease is not always painful, and many cases are asymptomatic [20, 21], it can be pretty disabling [22, 23]. It affects mainly men 25-45 years old [14, 15], with axial back pain that worsens when leaning forward, lifting weights, and getting in and out of the car [24, 25].

When medical treatments are ineffective [26 - 30], surgery may be helpful [31, 32]. The standard treatment, lumbar arthrodesis (fusion) [31, 33], can be performed through anterior or posterior approaches [31, 34 - 38]. On the one hand, posterior lumbar fusion disrupts paraspinal musculature [39 - 42], causing chronic pain and functional impairment [40, 43]. On the other hand, anterior lumbar arthrodesis avoids paraspinal muscle damage [42] but risks abdominal vessel injury and retrograde ejaculation [44 - 46].

Moreover, lumbar fusion can induce pseudoarthrosis [47, 48], adjoining level overloading [49, 50] with facet joint arthritis [51, 52], and disc degeneration [53 - 55]. Consequently, a reoperation to extend the arthrodesis is not uncommon [50, 56] in a term that varies depending on the number of fused levels [35, 50, 51, 57].

Schellnäck and Büttner-Janz [58] in the 1980s implanted the first total lumbar disc prosthesis, but the first implants had many problems [59 - 61], minimized through a continuous improvement (Charitè) [62] and the introduction of new designs [63] (Prodisc™ [64, 65], Activ-L™ [66, 67], Maverick-L™ [68, 69], Cadisc-L™ [70], Baguera-L™ [71], M6-L™ [72]).

Many studies comparing lumbar arthrodesis *versus* arthroplasty [73 - 82] report that with the latter, there is a higher percentage of return to the same job post [75, 83], a better quality of life [84, 85], a lower incidence of the adjoining level syndrome [73, 74, 77, 86] and a lower number of reoperations [80]. However, total disc prosthesis induces facet joint arthritis of the operated [87 - 89] and the supra-adjoining levels [88, 90 - 92] with chronic low back pain [93]. This degenerative process correlates with the excessive mobility of the total disc prostheses [94 - 96]. It is more evident in those with a greater motion range (Charitè) [97, 98] and when the rotation center is not in the posterior third of the intervertebral disc (Prodisc™ [99], Activ-L™ [100]).

Symptoms that make a Total Disc Prosthesis an Option

The usual complaints are low back pain radiating anteriorly to the groin and genital area at times, affecting one or both sides [101]. When there is also nerve root compression, patients may complain of leg pain [102], but waist pain is usually the most prevalent [103]. Low back pain worsens when bending forward, standing up from leaning forward, and lifting weights. Therefore, a total lumbar disc prosthesis is an option if the dominant feature is back pain with this clinical characteristic [104].

Not all patients are susceptible to a lumbar disc prosthesis. Solid bones are generally required, so osteoporosis is a contraindication. Otherwise, the prosthesis may sink into the vertebral body.

If there is facet joint arthritis, the disc prosthesis is not indicated because motion preservation will be at the price of significant lower back pain.

Inclusion Criteria

• Patients should be included between 18 and 50 years of age since, above that age, there is usually facet joint arthritis.

• Chronic lower back pain with or without leg pain originating from degenerated discs and with no signs of lumbar facet joint arthritis.

• Discogenic lower back pain that worsens in flexion but not in extension and has a truncal distribution with possible anterior irradiation towards the groins or genital area.

• MRI findings compatible with lumbar disc disease.

• No vertebral instability or listhesis of the levels in plain X-ray studies.

• No response to 6 weeks of conservative, non-surgical treatment or symptom progression.

• No previous treatment, such as microdiscectomy, laminectomy, or lumbar arthrodesis.

Intervertebral disc degeneration was measured with the Modic [106, 107] scale grade II or III [58, 105].

No facet joint osteoarthritis evaluated with the Fujiwara [108] and Pathria [109] scales.

Exclusion Criteria

• Facet joint arthropathy.

• Spine deformity or instability.

• Spinal canal stenosis.

• Previous spine fracture.

• Mobile spondylolisthesis of > 2 mm of translation and/or more than 11° of angular in flexion-extension standing up plain x-ray studies.

• Osteoporosis.

• Spinal metastases.

• A metabolic bone disease that may interfere with the implant or surgical procedure.

• Rheumatoid arthritis, lupus, or other autoimmune diseases affecting the musculoskeletal system.

• Other conditions or anatomical alterations which make the anterior surgical approach to the lumbar spine unfeasible.

• Allergy to stainless steel, titanium, or its alloys.

• Fixed or permanent neurological deficit.

• Active systemic infection or infection at the surgical site, including HIV and hepatitis C.

• Drug or alcohol abuse.

• Obesity (body mass index [BMI] >35) [110].

Types of Total Lumbar Disc Prosthesis

We can group them as the elastomeric and the ball and socket.

The elastomeric group has an elastomeric core (M6-L™, Spinal Kinetics, Sunnyvale, California, EUA; Cadisc-L™, Ranier Technology, Cambridge, United Kingdom; Freedom Lumbar Disc™, Axiomed Spine, Cleveland, OH, EUA) (Fig. **1**).

ELASTOMERIC TOTAL LUMBAR DISC PROSTHESES

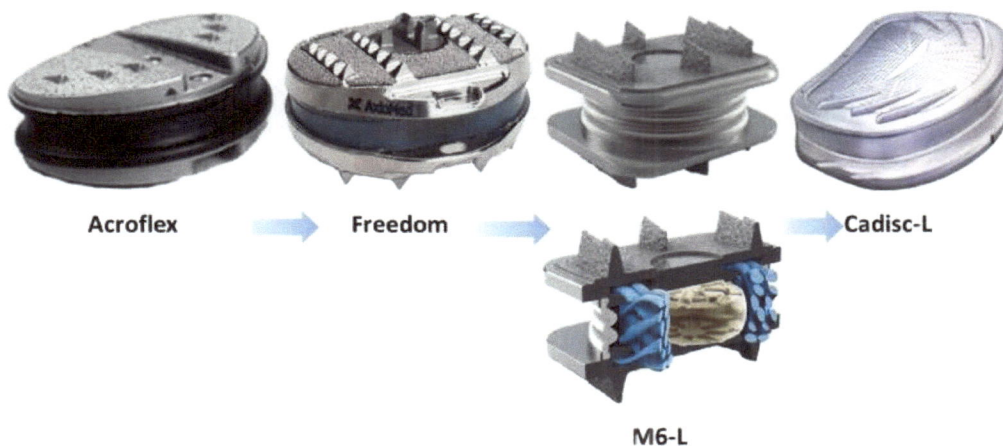

Fig. (1). Elastomeric total lumbar disc prosthesis.

The ball and socket implants are composed of three elements: two metal plates and an intermediate piece. This piece can move freely (SB III Charitè™, DePuy Spine, Inc., Raynham, MA, EE. UU.), in a semi-constrained fashion (ProDisc-L™, Synthes Spine, West Chester, NY, EE. UU.; Activ-L™, Aesculap, Tütlingen, Alemania; Baguera™, Spineart, Ginebra, Suiza) or not move at all (Maverick™, Medtronic SofamorDanek, Inc., Memphis, TN, EE. UU.). Mobile core devices (Charitè III™) induce facet joint overload in extension and can fasten degeneration [111]. Fixed centerpiece prostheses (Maverick ™) do not overload these joints as much, but as their rotation center is fixed [112], they do not reproduce the intact disc kinematics [113]. Another factor to consider is that the facet joint pressure increases in flexion, extension, and lateral flexion proportional to the decrease in the artificial lumbar disc articular surface radius and decreases in axial rotation [95]. This radius is the largest for SB Charitè™ and Prodisc L™, intermediate for Activ-L™ and Baguera™, and minimal for Maverick™ (Fig. **2**).

SURGICAL PROCEDURE

The surgical incision varies according to the disc level (Fig. **3**).

BALL AND SOCKET TOTAL LUMBAR DISC REPLACEMENT

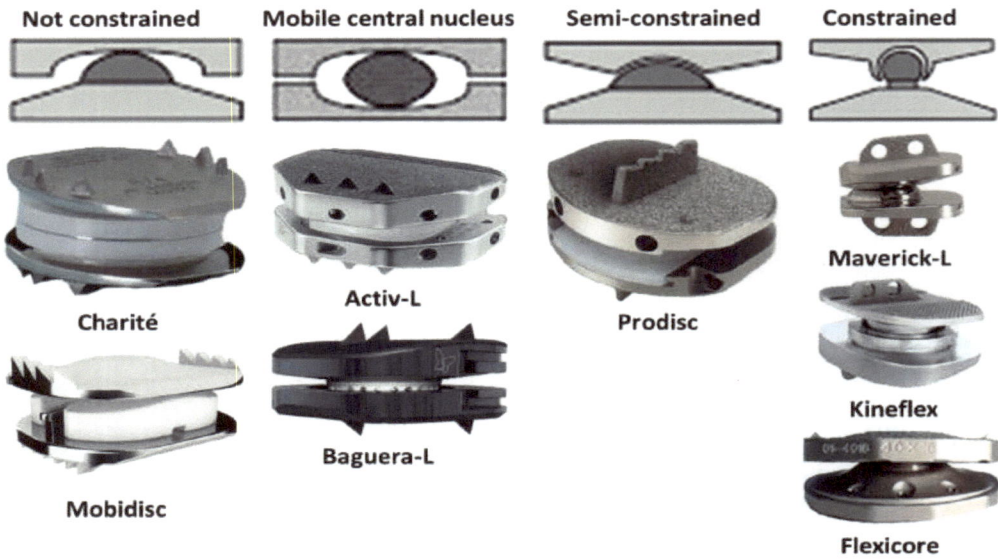

Fig. (2). Ball and socket total lumbar disc prostheses.

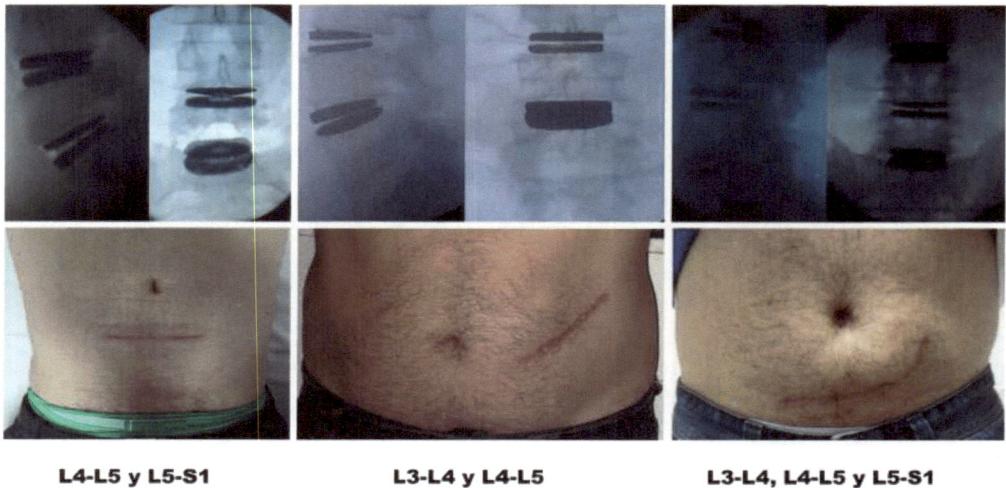

Fig. (3). Types of skin incisions for surgical insertion of total lumbar disc prostheses.

The anterior approach to the lumbar spine is made through a midline or a paramedian skin incision. For the L_4-L_5 and L_5-S_1, we favor a horizontal midline incision. The anterior rectus fascia is opened in a craniocaudal direction, and the muscle is elevated, exposing the posterior fascia of this muscle. This fascia is opened laterally, and the peritoneal contents are moved medially, reaching the retroperitoneal space. The ureter must be separated bluntly together with the peritoneum. Dissection proceeds depending on the disc once the great abdominal vessels are identified. To reach L_5-S_1, the iliac vessels arteries and veins are dissected carefully, and the mid-sacral artery is coagulated and cut to expose the vena cava end at the crotch where both iliac veins reach it. To avoid unintentional hypogastric plexus damage, we recommend careful dissection and hemostasis with bipolar coagulation. Next, the anterior part of the L_5-S_1 annulus and the nucleus pulposus are removed. If a discal hernia is inside the spinal canal, it is possible to recover the herniated discal fragment and remove it under magnification with loupes. Then, the space is measured to decide which total disc implant size and height will be required and the corresponding prosthesis inserted. The bed must be completely flat to prevent wrong implant insertion (Fig. **4**).

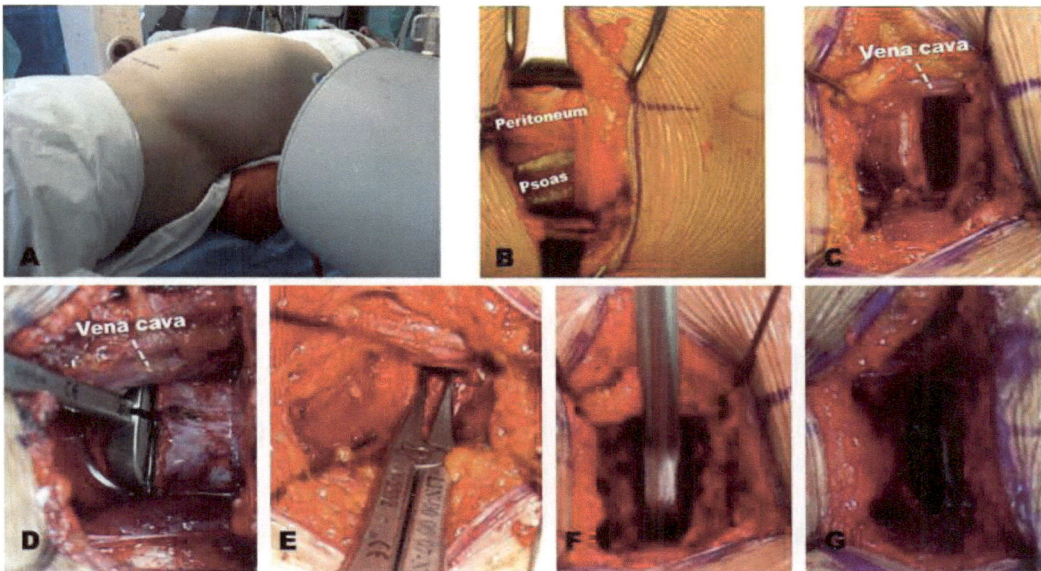

Fig. (4). Steps in L_5-S_1 total lumbar disc prosthesis.

With an AP X-ray, we will ensure the implant is centered in the midline, no more than 5mm from the midline. The asymmetrical insertion will induce abnormal biomechanics with increased subsidence risk and facet joint overload. Finally, a plain lateral x-ray confirms the rear implant part is no more than 4mm from the posterior vertebral body border (Fig. **5**). The lumbar disc prosthesis should be in its ideal position to reduce the facet joint overload [114, 115].

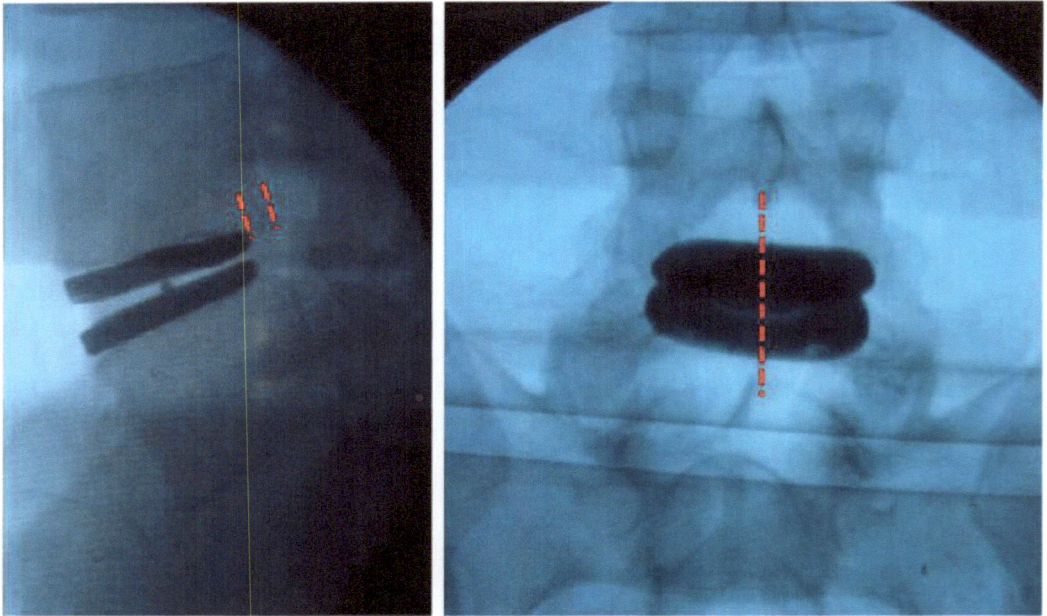

Fig. (5). Ideal total lumbar disc placement.

In the case of the L_4-L_5 disc, the first surgical maneuver, once the vena cava is exposed, is looking for a vein coming from the abdominal wall at the L_4-L_5 disc level on the lateral aspect. This vein tethers the vena cava and prevents displacement in a medial direction. Indeed, this vein may be avulsed from the vena cava if dissection is not done carefully, resulting in a copious hemorrhage. Also, suturing the hole in such a deep surgical wound is not easy. Thus, the best attitude is to look for this abdominal wall vein and ligate and dissect it. Then, the vena cava is no longer tethered and can be easily displaced in a medial direction. The next step is to expose the L_4-L_5 anterior annulus and remove it with the nucleus pulposus. Compared to the L_5-S_1 disc, perfect midline implant insertion is technically more difficult because the aorta and vena cava can make the procedure difficult. However, the implant must have the maximum possible size, an adequate height, and be placed centered A.P. and no more than 4mm from the posterior vertebral body border.

Higher levels need a more lateral skin incision. Finally, the retroperitoneal space is reached at the Spiegel line, lateral to the anterior rectus muscle. Then, the steps are the same as previously mentioned, but the L_4-L_5 abdominal wall vein does not need to be ligated.

Risks Involved in Total Disc Replacement

When artificial discs are implanted, complications are like those associated with anterior spinal fusion. These complications include, among others: infection, great abdominal vessel or nerve injury, prosthetic disc dislocation, rupture or subsidence (Figs. **6** and **7**), implant wear and tear, persistent low back pain, radicular pain, retrograde ejaculation, vaginal dryness, bladder incontinence and death (mainly due to catastrophic blood loss due to serious great abdominal vessel injury).

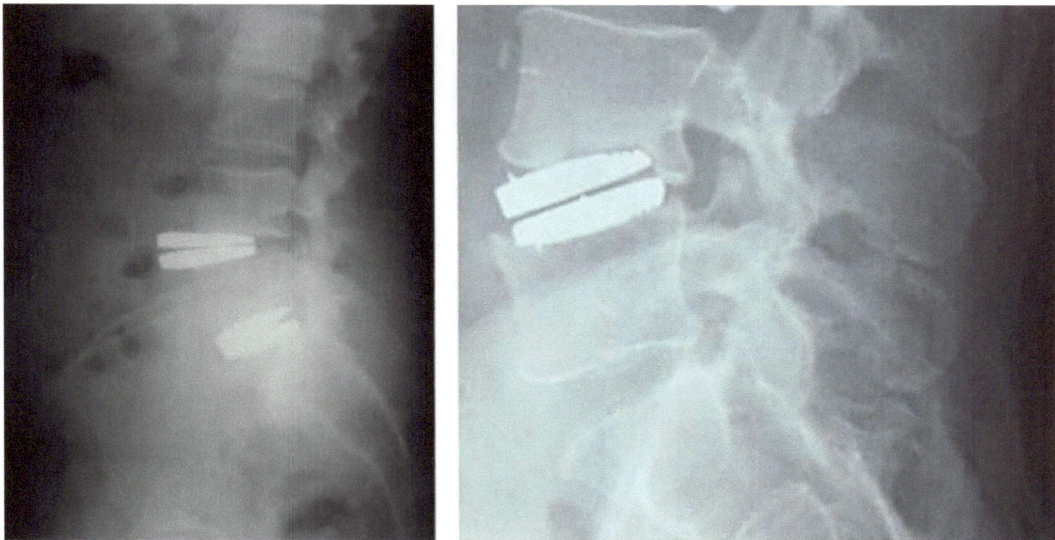

Extrusion   **Subsidence**

Fig. (6). Total lumbar disc prosthesis extrusion and subsidence.

Problems with the Total Disc Prostheses

In the elastomeric group, the main risk is that its core may undergo degeneration [116] as with other models, forcing their withdrawal from the market (Acroflex™, Acromed Corporation, Cleveland, OH, EE. UU.) [117, 118].

The problems with the ball and socket prosthesis are [95]:

- The inability to reproduce the intact spine kinematic and biomechanical characteristics [95, 119] induces non-physiologic loads for ligaments, muscles, and facet joints [120 - 125], leading to poor clinical outcomes [88, 90, 119].
- Excessive motion range, particularly in axial rotation [97], must be limited by muscles, ligaments, and facet joints, with long-term degenerative changes [110,

114]. Facet joint arthritis is among the most common causes of lumbar disc arthroplasty failure [90, 96, 126].

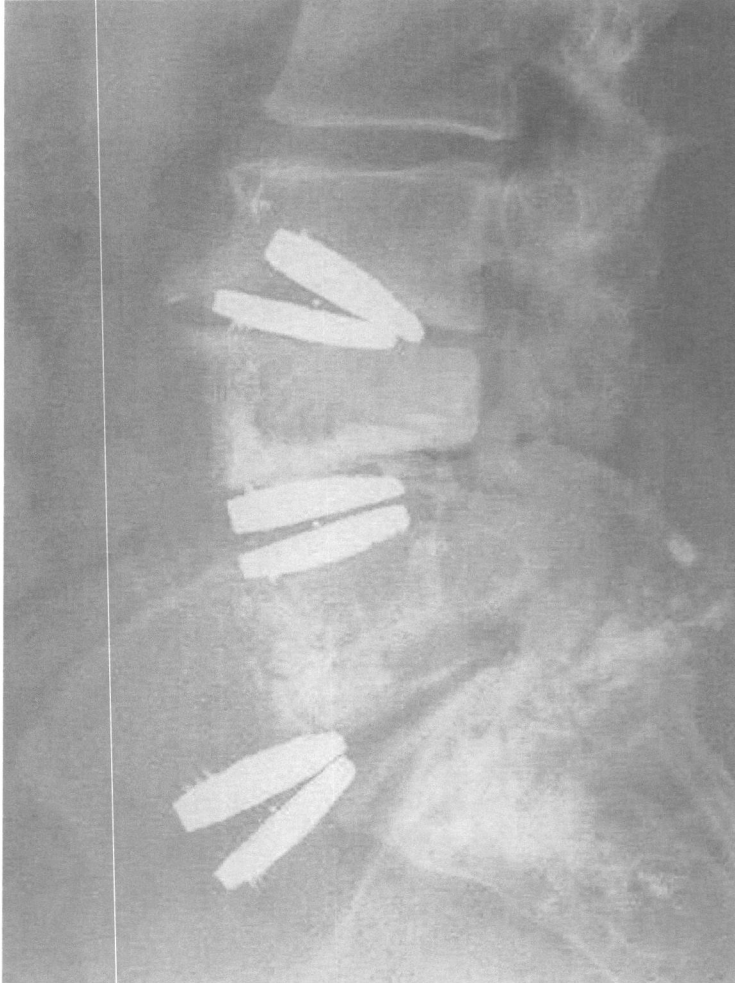

Fig. (7). Extrusion and subsidence in a patient with osteoporosis.

- Implant subsidence inside the endplates [59, 120, 124, 127 - 130]. The implant must be wide enough to transmit the load to the endplate's ring apophysis. Osteoporosis facilitates the occurrence of this problem.
- Dislocation or migration [59, 120, 121, 124, 129 - 137], more frequent with freely moving inlay devices (Charitè™) [59, 124, 136, 138, 139], but also in absent middle piece prostheses (Maverick™) [131]. Implant oversize also facilitates this problem [114].

- Wear, tear, and deformation [120, 130, 140 - 143]. The metallic and plastic particles induce a local inflammatory reaction with osteolysis [128, 142], facilitating implant loosening, migration, and subsidence [144, 145]. The amount of debris is more significant in prostheses with an ultra-high molecular weight polyethylene (UHMWPE) intermediate piece (Charitè™, Prodisc L™, Activ L™, Baguera™) [142, 146] and less with metal-on-metal prostheses (Maverick™) [147]. Still, the released metal ions can induce systemic reactions, particularly in those made of cobalt-chromium-molybdenum (CoCr28Mo6 alloy) [148]. The solution is to cover the articular surfaces with high-temperature treated carbon ("diamond-like carbon") (Baguera™) [71].

The ideal would be a lumbar disc prosthesis reproducing the intact spine's movements and mobility range, minimizing further wear rates, and having shock absorption capacity. Therefore, we designed a new CoCr28Mo6 metal-metal alloy lumbar disc prosthesis in this venue. It has two metallic plates made of CoCr28Mo6 alloy and a ring-shaped intermediate piece made of polycarbonate urethane (PCU) to improve load transmission and allow shock absorption (HELIYON-D-22-15268R3, ADDISC LUMBAR DISC PROSTHESIS: ANALYTICAL AND FEA TESTING OF NOVEL IMPLANTS).

Another critical aspect is removing the anterior part of the intervertebral disc annulus when implanting the total lumbar disc prosthesis [149 - 151]. As this part of the annulus limits the movement range in extension and axial rotation [152], the immediate post-operative result is excess mobility, especially in extension and axial rotation [94 - 96]. Unfortunately, this causes facet joint overload, with consequent arthritis [153]. Repairing the anterior part of the annulus during the surgical procedure is under debate [154]. From the outset, the technique is not easy [155] because it limits the space for the lumbar disc prosthesis, and if it is not large enough to transmit the load to the ring apophysis, it may sink into the vertebral endplates ("subsidence) [127]. On the other hand, re-anchoring the anterior part of the annulus to the vertebral endplates presents severe technical problems.

The general idea is that post-operative healing will gradually reduce the excess mobility allowed by the lumbar disc prosthesis and that it will have a range of motion that will approximate that of an intact intervertebral disc. However, this empirical idea has never been shown to have any objective basis.

Goals with Total Disc Prostheses

- Maintain spine movement.

- Relieve pain and maintain activity.

• Restore the intervertebral disc's height and the spine's physiological curvature.

• Reduce recovery time after the surgical procedure.

• Minimize adjoining level overload and subsequent degeneration.

What Happens after the Surgical Procedure?

Recovery is quick, and the biggest problem is the discomfort from the incision in the abdominal wall (such as a cesarean section) [105]. Generally, the patient's mobilization is early, and the return to work is usually quick. The complications are those of any surgical intervention: pain, infection, hemorrhage, and root damage. Two specific risks are vascular injury (due to the surgical handling of the great abdominal vessels) and retrograde ejaculation or vaginal dryness. In this case, ejaculation occurs inside the urinary bladder and not outside. It is rare but can occur in 5% of cases. Wearing a belt is unnecessary postoperatively, but a gradual re-incorporation to normal activities is recommended, avoiding those involving spine extension.

CONCLUSION

Motion preservation is advisable to maintain spinal biomechanics and avoid adjacent-level degeneration. The different total disc prosthesis designs provide different movement ranges and thus must be considered when selecting the most appropriate for the individual patient. Ideal total disc prosthesis implantation prevents unwanted spinal biomechanics and provides the best clinical results.

REFERENCES

[1] Fatoye F, Gebrye T, Odeyemi I. Real-world incidence and prevalence of low back pain using routinely collected data. Rheumatol Int 2019; 39(4): 619-26.
[http://dx.doi.org/10.1007/s00296-019-04273-0] [PMID: 30848349]

[2] Meucci RD, Fassa AG, Faria NMX. Prevalence of chronic low back pain: systematic review. Rev Saude Publica 2015; 49(0): 1-15.
[http://dx.doi.org/10.1590/S0034-8910.2015049005874] [PMID: 26487293]

[3] Manchikanti L, Singh V, Falco FJE, Benyamin RM, Hirsch JA. Epidemiology of low back pain in adults. Neuromodulation 2014; 17 (Suppl. 2): 3-10.
[http://dx.doi.org/10.1111/ner.12018] [PMID: 25395111]

[4] Urits I, Burshtein A, Sharma M, *et al.* Low back pain, a comprehensive review: pathophysiology, diagnosis, and treatment. Curr Pain Headache Rep 2019; 23(3): 23-7.
[http://dx.doi.org/10.1007/s11916-019-0757-1] [PMID: 30854609]

[5] Buchbinder R, van Tulder M, Öberg B, *et al.* Low back pain: a call for action. Lancet 2018; 391(10137): 2384-8.
[http://dx.doi.org/10.1016/S0140-6736(18)30488-4] [PMID: 29573871]

[6] Hartvigsen J, Hancock MJ, Kongsted A, *et al.* What low back pain is and why we need to pay attention. Lancet 2018; 391(10137): 2356-67.

[http://dx.doi.org/10.1016/S0140-6736(18)30480-X] [PMID: 29573870]

[7]   Clark S, Horton R. Low back pain: a major global challenge. Lancet 2018; 391(10137): 2302-10.
        [http://dx.doi.org/10.1016/S0140-6736(18)30725-6] [PMID: 29573869]

[8]   Yang H, Haldeman S, Lu ML, Baker D. Low back pain prevalence and related workplace
        psychosocial risk factors: a study using data from the 2010 national health interview survey. J
        Manipulative Physiol Ther 2016; 39(7): 459-72.
        [http://dx.doi.org/10.1016/j.jmpt.2016.07.004] [PMID: 27568831]

[9]   Luckhaupt SE, Dahlhamer JM, Gonzales GT, Lu ML, Groenewold M, Sweeney MH, *et al.* Prevalence,
        recognition of work-relatedness, and effect on work of low back pain among U.S. workers. Ann Intern
        Med 2019; 20(171(4)): 301-4.

[10]   Becker BA, Childress MA. Nonspecific low back pain and return to work. Am Fam Physician 2019;
        100(11): 697-703.
        [PMID: 31790184]

[11]   Jess MA, Hamilton S, Ryan CG, Wellburn S, Martin D. Exploring the origin of low back pain sub-
        classification: a scoping review protocol. JBI Database Syst Rev Implement Reports 2019; 17(8):
        1600-6.
        [http://dx.doi.org/10.11124/JBISRIR-2017-003805] [PMID: 30889071]

[12]   MacDonald J, Stuart E, Rodenberg R. Musculoskeletal Low Back Pain in School-aged Children.
        JAMA Pediatr 2017; 171(3): 280-7.
        [http://dx.doi.org/10.1001/jamapediatrics.2016.3334] [PMID: 28135365]

[13]   Riihimäki H. Low-back pain, its origin and risk indicators. Scand J Work Environ Health 1991; 17(2):
        81-90.
        [http://dx.doi.org/10.5271/sjweh.1728] [PMID: 1828614]

[14]   Schwertner DS, Oliveira RANS, Koerich MHAL, Motta AF, Pimenta AL, Gioda FR. Prevalence of
        low back pain in young Brazilians and associated factors: Sex, physical activity, sedentary behavior,
        sleep and body mass index. J Back Musculoskeletal Rehabil 2020; 33(2): 233-44.
        [http://dx.doi.org/10.3233/BMR-170821] [PMID: 31356188]

[15]   Hyodo H, Sato T, Sasaki H, Tanaka Y. Discogenic pain in acute nonspecific low-back pain. Eur Spine
        J 2005; 14(6): 573-7.
        [http://dx.doi.org/10.1007/s00586-004-0844-8] [PMID: 15668774]

[16]   Grabovac I, Dorner TE. Association between low back pain and various everyday performances. Wien
        Klin Wochenschr 2019; 131(21-22): 541-9.
        [http://dx.doi.org/10.1007/s00508-019-01542-7] [PMID: 31493101]

[17]   Müller CF, Monrad T, Biering-Sørensen F, Darre E, Deis A, Kryger P. The influence of previous low
        back trouble, general health, and working conditions on future sick-listing because of low back
        trouble. A 15-year follow-up study of risk indicators for self-reported sick-listing caused by low back
        trouble. Spine 1999; 24(15): 1562-70.
        [http://dx.doi.org/10.1097/00007632-199908010-00010] [PMID: 10457576]

[18]   Bartys S, Frederiksen P, Bendix T, Burton K. System influences on work disability due to low back
        pain: An international evidence synthesis. Health Policy 2017; 121(8): 903-12.
        [http://dx.doi.org/10.1016/j.healthpol.2017.05.011] [PMID: 28595897]

[19]   Geurts JW, Willems PC, Kallewaard JW, van Kleef M, Dirksen C. The impact of chronic discogenic
        low back pain: costs and patients' burden. Pain Res Manag 2018; 2018: 1-8.
        [http://dx.doi.org/10.1155/2018/4696180] [PMID: 30364097]

[20]   Boos N, Semmer N, Elfering A, *et al.* Natural history of individuals with asymptomatic disc
        abnormalities in magnetic resonance imaging: predictors of low back pain-related medical consultation
        and work incapacity. Spine 2000; 25(12): 1484-92.
        [http://dx.doi.org/10.1097/00007632-200006150-00006] [PMID: 10851096]

[21] Middendorp M, Vogl TJ, Kollias K, Kafchitsas K, Khan MF, Maataoui A. Association between intervertebral disc degeneration and the Oswestry Disability Index. J Back Musculoskeletal Rehabil 2017; 30(4): 819-23.
[http://dx.doi.org/10.3233/BMR-150516] [PMID: 28372314]

[22] Simon J, McAuliffe M, Shamim F, Vuong N, Tahaei A. Discogenic low back pain. Phys Med Rehabil Clin N Am 2014; 25(2): 305-17.
[http://dx.doi.org/10.1016/j.pmr.2014.01.006] [PMID: 24787335]

[23] Zhao L, Manchikanti L, Kaye AD, Abd-Elsayed A. Treatment of discogenic low back pain: current treatment strategies and future options—a literature review. Curr Pain Headache Rep 2019; 23(11): 86.
[http://dx.doi.org/10.1007/s11916-019-0821-x] [PMID: 31707499]

[24] Chan AYP, Ford JJ, McMeeken JM, Wilde VE. Preliminary evidence for the features of non-reducible discogenic low back pain: survey of an international physiotherapy expert panel with the Delphi technique. Physiotherapy 2013; 99(3): 212-20.
[http://dx.doi.org/10.1016/j.physio.2012.09.007] [PMID: 23517665]

[25] Nyström B, Weber H, Schillberg B, Taube A. Symptoms and signs possibly indicating segmental, discogenic pain. A fusion study with 18 years of follow-up. Scand J Pain 2017; 16(1): 213-20.
[http://dx.doi.org/10.1016/j.sjpain.2016.10.007] [PMID: 28850405]

[26] Helm S, Simopoulos TT, Stojanovic M, Abdi S, El Terany MA. Effectiveness of thermal annular procedures in treating discogenic low back pain. Pain Physician 2017; 6(20;6): 447-70.
[http://dx.doi.org/10.36076/ppj/447] [PMID: 28934777]

[27] Manchikanti L, Pampati V, Kaye AD, Hirsch JA. Therapeutic lumbar facet joint nerve blocks in the treatment of chronic low back pain: cost utility analysis based on a randomized controlled trial. Korean J Pain 2018; 31(1): 27-38.
[http://dx.doi.org/10.3344/kjp.2018.31.1.27] [PMID: 29372023]

[28] Zeckser J, Wolff M, Tucker J, Goodwin J. Multipotent mesenchymal stem cell treatment for discogenic low back pain and disc degeneration. Stem Cells Int 2016; 2016(1): 3908389.
[http://dx.doi.org/10.1155/2016/3908389] [PMID: 26880958]

[29] Karimi A, Mahmoudzadeh A, Rezaeian ZS, Dommerholt J. The effect of dry needling on the radiating pain in subjects with discogenic low-back pain: A randomized control trial. J Res Med Sci 2016; 21(1): 86.
[http://dx.doi.org/10.4103/1735-1995.192502] [PMID: 28163732]

[30] Rahimzadeh P, Imani F, Ghahremani M, Faiz SHR. Comparison of percutaneous intradiscal ozone injection with laser disc decompression in discogenic low back pain. J Pain Res 2018; 11: 1405-10.
[http://dx.doi.org/10.2147/JPR.S164335] [PMID: 30104895]

[31] Mobbs RJ, Phan K, Malham G, Seex K, Rao PJ. Lumbar interbody fusion: techniques, indications and comparison of interbody fusion options including PLIF, TLIF, MI-TLIF, OLIF/ATP, LLIF and ALIF. J Spine Surg 2015; 1(1): 2-18.
[PMID: 27683674]

[32] Willems P. Decision making in surgical treatment of chronic low back pain: the performance of prognostic tests to select patients for lumbar spinal fusion. Acta Orthop 2013; 84(sup349): 1-37.
[http://dx.doi.org/10.3109/17453674.2012.753565] [PMID: 23427903]

[33] Bydon M, De la Garza-Ramos R, Macki M, Baker A, Gokaslan AK, Bydon A. Lumbar fusion *versus* nonoperative management for treatment of discogenic low back pain: a systematic review and meta-analysis of randomized controlled trials. J Spinal Disord Tech 2014; 27(5): 297-304.
[http://dx.doi.org/10.1097/BSD.0000000000000072] [PMID: 24346052]

[34] Hara M, Nishimura Y, Nakajima Y, *et al.* Transforaminal lumbar interbody fusion for lumbar degenerative disorders: mini-open TLIF and corrective TLIF. Neurol Med Chir (Tokyo) 2015; 55(7): 547-56.

[http://dx.doi.org/10.2176/nmc.oa.2014-0402] [PMID: 26119895]

[35] Louie PK, Varthi AG, Narain AS, *et al*. Stand-alone lateral lumbar interbody fusion for the treatment of symptomatic adjacent segment degeneration following previous lumbar fusion. Spine J 2018; 18(11): 2025-32.
[http://dx.doi.org/10.1016/j.spinee.2018.04.008] [PMID: 29679730]

[36] Ni J, Fang X, Zhong W, Liu N, Wood KB. Anterior lumbar interbody fusion for degenerative discogenic low back pain. Medicine (Baltimore) 2015; 94(43): e1851.
[http://dx.doi.org/10.1097/MD.0000000000001851] [PMID: 26512594]

[37] Duan X, Shao Z, Xie K, Wang Z. Research progress of percutaneous 360 degree axial lumbar interbody fusion technique. Zhongguo Xiu Fu Chong Jian Wai Ke Za Zhi. 2009 Aug;23(8):917-20. Chinese.
[PMID: 19728605]

[38] Edgard-Rosa G, Geneste G, Nègre G, Marnay T. Midline anterior approach from the right side to the lumbar spine for interbody fusion and total disc replacement: a new mobilization technique of the vena cava. Spine 2012; 37(9): E562-9.
[http://dx.doi.org/10.1097/BRS.0b013e31823a0a87] [PMID: 22517482]

[39] Cha JR, Kim YC, Yoon WK, *et al*. The recovery of damaged paraspinal muscles by posterior surgical treatment for patients with lumbar degenerative diseases and its clinical consequence. J Back Musculoskeletal Rehabil 2017; 30(4): 801-9.
[http://dx.doi.org/10.3233/BMR-150455] [PMID: 28372312]

[40] Waschke A, Hartmann C, Walter J, *et al*. Denervation and atrophy of paraspinal muscles after open lumbar interbody fusion is associated with clinical outcome—electromyographic and CT-volumetric investigation of 30 patients. Acta Neurochir (Wien) 2014; 156(2): 235-44.
[http://dx.doi.org/10.1007/s00701-013-1981-9] [PMID: 24384989]

[41] Gille O, Jolivet E, Dousset V, *et al*. Erector spinae muscle changes on magnetic resonance imaging following lumbar surgery through a posterior approach. Spine 2007; 32(11): 1236-41.
[http://dx.doi.org/10.1097/BRS.0b013e31805471fe] [PMID: 17495782]

[42] Motosuneya T, Asazuma T, Tsuji T, Watanabe H, Nakayama Y, Nemoto K. Postoperative change of the cross-sectional area of back musculature after 5 surgical procedures as assessed by magnetic resonance imaging. J Spinal Disord Tech 2006; 19(5): 318-22.
[http://dx.doi.org/10.1097/01.bsd.0000211205.15997.06] [PMID: 16826001]

[43] Tandon R, Kiyawat V, Kumar N. Clinical correlation between muscle damage and oswestry disability index score after open lumbar surgery: does open surgery reduces functional ability? Asian Spine J 2018; 12(3): 518-23.
[http://dx.doi.org/10.4184/asj.2018.12.3.518] [PMID: 29879780]

[44] Qureshi R, Puvanesarajah V, Jain A, Shimer AL, Shen FH, Hassanzadeh H. A comparison of anterior and posterior lumbar interbody fusions. Spine 2017; 42(24): 1865-70.
[http://dx.doi.org/10.1097/BRS.0000000000002248] [PMID: 28549000]

[45] Goz V, Weinreb JH, Schwab F, Lafage V, Errico TJ. Comparison of complications, costs, and length of stay of three different lumbar interbody fusion techniques: an analysis of the Nationwide Inpatient Sample database. Spine J 2014; 14(9): 2019-27.
[http://dx.doi.org/10.1016/j.spinee.2013.11.050] [PMID: 24333459]

[46] Fischer CR, Braaksma B, Peters A, *et al*. Outcomes and complications of the midline anterior approach 3 years after lumbar spine surgery. Adv Orthop 2014; 2014: 1-10.
[http://dx.doi.org/10.1155/2014/142604] [PMID: 25610657]

[47] Manzur M, Virk SS, Jivanelli B, *et al*. The rate of fusion for stand-alone anterior lumbar interbody fusion: a systematic review. Spine J 2019; 19(7): 1294-301.
[http://dx.doi.org/10.1016/j.spinee.2019.03.001] [PMID: 30872148]

[48]   Jaeger A, Giber D, Bastard C, *et al.* Risk factors of instrumentation failure and pseudarthrosis after stand-alone L5-S1 anterior lumbar interbody fusion: a retrospective cohort study. J Neurosurg Spine 2019; 31(3): 338-46.
        [PMID: 31151106]

[49]   Koenders N, Rushton A, Verra ML, Willems PC, Hoogeboom TJ, Staal JB. Pain and disability after first-time spinal fusion for lumbar degenerative disorders: a systematic review and meta-analysis. Eur Spine J 2019; 28(4): 696-709.
        [http://dx.doi.org/10.1007/s00586-018-5680-3] [PMID: 29995169]

[50]   Hashimoto K, Aizawa T, Kanno H, Itoi E. Adjacent segment degeneration after fusion spinal surgery—a systematic review. Int Orthop 2019; 43(4): 987-93.
        [http://dx.doi.org/10.1007/s00264-018-4241-z] [PMID: 30470865]

[51]   Ma Z, Huang S, Sun J, Li F, Sun J, Pi G. Risk factors for upper adjacent segment degeneration after multi-level posterior lumbar spinal fusion surgery. J Orthop Surg Res 2019; 14(1): 89.
        [http://dx.doi.org/10.1186/s13018-019-1126-9] [PMID: 30922408]

[52]   Ma J, Jia H, Ma X, *et al.* Evaluation of the stress distribution change at the adjacent facet joints after lumbar fusion surgery: A biomechanical study. Proc Inst Mech Eng H 2014; 228(7): 665-73.
        [http://dx.doi.org/10.1177/0954411914541435] [PMID: 24963037]

[53]   Michael AP, Weber MW, Delfino KR, Ganapathy V. Adjacent-segment disease following two-level axial lumbar interbody fusion. J Neurosurg Spine 19 de abril de 2019; 1-8.

[54]   Lee JC, Kim Y, Soh JW, Shin BJ. Risk factors of adjacent segment disease requiring surgery after lumbar spinal fusion: comparison of posterior lumbar interbody fusion and posterolateral fusion. Spine 2014; 39(5): E339-45.
        [http://dx.doi.org/10.1097/BRS.0000000000000164] [PMID: 24365899]

[55]   Ženčica P, Chaloupka R, Hladíková J, Krbec M. Adjacent segment degeneration after lumbosacral fusion in spondylolisthesis: a retrospective radiological and clinical analysis. Acta Chir Orthop Traumatol Cech 2010; 77(2): 124-30.
        [http://dx.doi.org/10.55095/achot2010/023] [PMID: 20447355]

[56]   Drysch A, Ajiboye RM, Sharma A, *et al.* Effectiveness of reoperations for adjacent segment disease following lumbar spinal fusion. Orthopedics 2018; 41(2): e161-7.
        [http://dx.doi.org/10.3928/01477447-20170621-02] [PMID: 28662247]

[57]   Zhong ZM, Deviren V, Tay B, Burch S, Berven SH. Adjacent segment disease after instrumented fusion for adult lumbar spondylolisthesis: Incidence and risk factors. Clin Neurol Neurosurg 2017; 156: 29-34.
        [http://dx.doi.org/10.1016/j.clineuro.2017.02.020] [PMID: 28288396]

[58]   Büttner-Janz K, Guyer RD, Ohnmeiss DD. Indications for lumbar total disc replacement: selecting the right patient with the right indication for the right total disc. Int J Spine Surg 2014; 8: 12.
        [http://dx.doi.org/10.14444/1012] [PMID: 25694946]

[59]   van Ooij A, Oner FC, Verbout AJ. Complications of artificial disc replacement: a report of 27 patients with the SB Charité disc. J Spinal Disord Tech 2003; 16(4): 369-83.
        [http://dx.doi.org/10.1097/00024720-200308000-00009] [PMID: 12902953]

[60]   Szpalski M, Gunzburg R, Mayer M. Spine arthroplasty: a historical review. Eur Spine J 2002; 11(S2) (Suppl. 2): S65-84.
        [http://dx.doi.org/10.1007/s00586-002-0474-y] [PMID: 12384726]

[61]   Bertagnoli R, Zigler J, Karg A, Voigt S. Complications and strategies for revision surgery in total disc replacement. Orthop Clin North Am 2005; 36(3): 389-95.
        [http://dx.doi.org/10.1016/j.ocl.2005.03.003] [PMID: 15950699]

[62]   Link HD. History, design and biomechanics of the LINK SB Charité artificial disc. Eur Spine J 2002; 11(S2) (Suppl. 2): S98-S105.

[http://dx.doi.org/10.1007/s00586-002-0475-x] [PMID: 12384729]

[63] Bono CM, Garfin SR. History and evolution of disc replacement. Spine J 2004; 4(6) (Suppl.): S145-50.
[http://dx.doi.org/10.1016/j.spinee.2004.07.005] [PMID: 15541659]

[64] Balderston JR, Gertz ZM, McIntosh T, Balderston RA. Long-term outcomes of 2-level total disc replacement using prodisc-L. Spine 2014; 39(11): 906-10.
[http://dx.doi.org/10.1097/BRS.0000000000000148] [PMID: 29504961]

[65] Park SJ, Lee CS, Chung SS, Lee KH, Kim WS, Lee JY. Long-term outcomes following lumbar total disc replacement using prodisc-II. Spine 2016; 41(11): 971-7.
[http://dx.doi.org/10.1097/BRS.0000000000001527] [PMID: 26909840]

[66] Austen S, Punt IM, Cleutjens JPM, *et al.* Clinical, radiological, histological and retrieval findings of Activ-L and Mobidisc total disc replacements: a study of two patients. Eur Spine J 2012; 21(S4) (Suppl. 4): 513-20.
[http://dx.doi.org/10.1007/s00586-011-2141-7] [PMID: 22245852]

[67] Lu S, Kong C, Hai Y, *et al.* Prospective clinical and radiographic results of activ L total disk replacement at 1- to 3-year follow-up. J Spinal Disord Tech 2015; 28(9): E544-50.
[http://dx.doi.org/10.1097/BSD.0000000000000237] [PMID: 25532603]

[68] Assaker R, Ritter-Lang K, Vardon D, *et al.* Maverick total disc replacement in a real-world patient population: a prospective, multicentre, observational study. Eur Spine J 2015; 24(9): 2047-55.
[http://dx.doi.org/10.1007/s00586-015-3918-x] [PMID: 26050106]

[69] Plais N, Thevenot X, Cogniet A, Rigal J, Le Huec JC. Maverick total disc arthroplasty performs well at 10 years follow-up: a prospective study with HRQL and balance analysis. Eur Spine J 2018; 27(3): 720-7.
[http://dx.doi.org/10.1007/s00586-017-5065-z] [PMID: 28382391]

[70] McNally D, Naylor J, Johnson S. An *in vitro* biomechanical comparison of CadiscTM-L with natural lumbar discs in axial compression and sagittal flexion. Eur Spine J Off Publ Eur Spine Soc Eur Spinal Deform Soc Eur Sect Cerv Spine Res Soc j 2012; 21(5): S612-617.

[71] Fransen P, Hansen-Algenstaedt N, Chatzisotiriou A, Noriega DCG, Pointillart V. Clinical results of cervical disc replacement with the Baguera C prosthesis after two years follow-up. Acta Orthop Belg 2018; 84(3): 345-51.
[PMID: 30840578]

[72] Schätz C, Ritter-Lang K, Gössel L, Dreßler N. Comparison of single-level and multiple-level outcomes of total disc arthroplasty: 24-month results. Int J Spine Surg 2015; 9: 14.
[http://dx.doi.org/10.14444/2014] [PMID: 26056629]

[73] Ding F, Jia Z, Zhao Z, *et al.* Total disc replacement *versus* fusion for lumbar degenerative disc disease: a systematic review of overlapping meta-analyses. Eur Spine J 2017; 26(3): 806-15.
[http://dx.doi.org/10.1007/s00586-016-4714-y] [PMID: 27448810]

[74] Bai D, Liang L, Zhang B, *et al.* Total disc replacement *versus* fusion for lumbar degenerative diseases - a meta-analysis of randomized controlled trials. Medicine (Baltimore) 2019; 98(29): e16460.
[http://dx.doi.org/10.1097/MD.0000000000016460] [PMID: 31335704]

[75] Guyer RD, McAfee PC, Banco RJ, *et al.* Prospective, randomized, multicenter Food and Drug Administration investigational device exemption study of lumbar total disc replacement with the CHARITÉ artificial disc *versus* lumbar fusion: Five-year follow-up. Spine J 2009; 9(5): 374-86.
[http://dx.doi.org/10.1016/j.spinee.2008.08.007] [PMID: 18805066]

[76] Panjabi M, Malcolmson G, Teng E, Tominaga Y, Henderson G, Serhan H. Hybrid testing of lumbar CHARITE discs *versus* fusions. Spine 2007; 32(9): 959-66.
[http://dx.doi.org/10.1097/01.brs.0000260792.13893.88] [PMID: 17450069]

[77] Gornet MF, Burkus JK, Dryer RF, Peloza JH, Schranck FW, Copay AG. Lumbar disc arthroplasty

versus anterior lumbar interbody fusion: 5-year outcomes for patients in the Maverick disc investigational device exemption study. J Neurosurg Spine 2019; 31(3): 347-56.
[http://dx.doi.org/10.3171/2019.2.SPINE181037] [PMID: 31100723]

[78]   Stubig T, Ahmed M, Ghasemi A, Nasto LA, Grevitt M. Total disc replacement *versus* anterior-posterior interbody fusion in the lumbar spine and lumbosacral junction: a cost analysis. Global Spine J 2018; 8(2): 129-36.
[http://dx.doi.org/10.1177/2192568217713009] [PMID: 29662742]

[79]   Li YZ, Sun P, Chen D, Tang L, Chen CH, Wu AM. Artificial total disc replacement *versus* fusion for lumbar degenerative disc disease: an update systematic review and meta-analysis. Turk Neurosurg 2020; 30(1): 1-10.
[PMID: 30984993]

[80]   Radcliff K, Spivak J, Darden B II, Janssen M, Bernard T, Zigler J. Five-year reoperation rates of 2-level lumbar total disk replacement *versus* fusion. Clin Spine Surg 2018; 31(1): 37-42.
[http://dx.doi.org/10.1097/BSD.0000000000000476] [PMID: 28005616]

[81]   Mattei TA, Beer J, Teles AR, Rehman AA, Aldag J, Dinh D. Clinical outcomes of total disc replacement *versus* anterior lumbar interbody fusion for surgical treatment of lumbar degenerative disc disease. Global Spine J 2017; 7(5): 452-9.
[http://dx.doi.org/10.1177/2192568217712714] [PMID: 28811990]

[82]   Berg S, Tullberg T, Branth B, Olerud C, Tropp H. Total disc replacement compared to lumbar fusion: a randomised controlled trial with 2-year follow-up. Eur Spine J 009; 18(10): 1512-9.

[83]   Guyer RD, Pettine K, Roh JS, *et al.* Five-year follow-up of a prospective, randomized trial comparing two lumbar total disc replacements. Spine 2016; 41(1): 3-8.
[http://dx.doi.org/10.1097/BRS.0000000000001168] [PMID: 26335669]

[84]   Clavel P, Ungureanu G, Catalá I, Montes G, Málaga X, Ríos M. Health-related quality of life in patients undergoing lumbar total disc replacement: A comparison with the general population. Clin Neurol Neurosurg 2017; 160: 119-24.
[http://dx.doi.org/10.1016/j.clineuro.2017.07.007] [PMID: 28719872]

[85]   Cui XD, Li HT, Zhang W, Zhang LL, Luo ZP, Yang HL. Mid- to long-term results of total disc replacement for lumbar degenerative disc disease: a systematic review. J Orthop Surg Res 2018; 13(1): 326.
[http://dx.doi.org/10.1186/s13018-018-1032-6] [PMID: 30585142]

[86]   Zigler J, Gornet MF, Ferko N, Cameron C, Schranck FW, Patel L. Comparison of lumbar total disc replacement with surgical spinal fusion for the treatment of single-level degenerative disc disease: A meta-analysis of 5-year outcomes from randomized controlled trials. Global Spine J 2018; 8(4): 413-23.
[http://dx.doi.org/10.1177/2192568217737317] [PMID: 29977727]

[87]   Shin MH, Ryu KS, Rathi NK, Park CK. Segmental translation after lumbar total disc replacement using Prodisc-L®: associated factors and relation to facet arthrosis. J Neurosurg Sci 2017; 61(1): 14-21.
[PMID: 25649063]

[88]   Botolin S, Puttlitz C, Baldini T, *et al.* Facet joint biomechanics at the treated and adjacent levels after total disc replacement. Spine 2011; 36(1): E27-32.
[http://dx.doi.org/10.1097/BRS.0b013e3181d2d071] [PMID: 20975623]

[89]   Shin MH, Ryu KS, Hur JW, Kim JS, Park CK. Association of facet tropism and progressive facet arthrosis after lumbar total disc replacement using ProDisc-L®. Eur Spine J 2013; 22(8): 1717-22.
[http://dx.doi.org/10.1007/s00586-012-2606-3] [PMID: 23291784]

[90]   Hu X, Li K. Stress changes of upper lumbar facet joint after discectomy and artificial disc replacement. Zhongguo Xiu Fu Chong Jian Wai Ke Za Zhi. 2005 Jun;19(6):427-30. Chinese.
[PMID: 16038454]

[91]   Park CK, Ryu KS, Jee WH. Degenerative changes of discs and facet joints in lumbar total disc replacement using ProDisc II: minimum two-year follow-up. Spine 2008; 33(16): 1755-61.
[http://dx.doi.org/10.1097/BRS.0b013e31817b8fed] [PMID: 18580548]

[92]   Siepe CJ, Zelenkov P, Sauri-Barraza JC, *et al.* The fate of facet joint and adjacent level disc degeneration following total lumbar disc replacement: a prospective clinical, X-ray, and magnetic resonance imaging investigation. Spine 2010; 35(22): 1991-2003.
[http://dx.doi.org/10.1097/BRS.0b013e3181d6f878] [PMID: 20881662]

[93]   Hellum C, Berg L, Gjertsen Ø, *et al.* Adjacent level degeneration and facet arthropathy after disc prosthesis surgery or rehabilitation in patients with chronic low back pain and degenerative disc: second report of a randomized study. Spine 2012; 37(25): 2063-73.
[http://dx.doi.org/10.1097/BRS.0b013e318263cc46] [PMID: 22706091]

[94]   Huang RC, Girardi FP, Cammisa FP Jr, Wright TM. The implications of constraint in lumbar total disc replacement. J Spinal Disord Tech 2003; 16(4): 412-7.
[http://dx.doi.org/10.1097/00024720-200308000-00014] [PMID: 12902958]

[95]   Choi J, Shin DA, Kim S. Biomechanical effects of the geometry of ball-and-socket artificial disc on lumbar spine. Spine 2017; 42(6): E332-9.
[http://dx.doi.org/10.1097/BRS.0000000000001789] [PMID: 27428389]

[96]   Schmidt H, Galbusera F, Rohlmann A, Zander T, Wilke HJ. Effect of multilevel lumbar disc arthroplasty on spine kinematics and facet joint loads in flexion and extension: a finite element analysis. Eur Spine J 2012; 21(S5) (Suppl. 5): 663-74.
[http://dx.doi.org/10.1007/s00586-010-1382-1] [PMID: 20361341]

[97]   Choi JI, Kim SH, Lim DJ, Ha SK, Kim SD. Biomechanical changes in disc pressure and facet strain after lumbar spinal arthroplasty with charité™ in the human cadaveric spine under physiologic compressive follower preload. Turk Neurosurg 2017; 27(2): 252-8.
[PMID: 27337240]

[98]   SariAli E, Lemaire JP, Pascal-Mousselard H, Carrier H, Skalli W. *In vivo* study of the kinematics in axial rotation of the lumbar spine after total intervertebral disc replacement: long-term results: a 10–14 years follow up evaluation. Eur Spine J 2006; 15(10): 1501-10.
[http://dx.doi.org/10.1007/s00586-005-0016-5]

[99]   Rohlmann A, Zander T, Bergmann G. Effect of total disc replacement with ProDisc on intersegmental rotation of the lumbar spine. Spine 1 de abril de 2005; 30(7): 738-43.
[http://dx.doi.org/10.1097/01.brs.0000157413.72276.c4]

[100] Zander T, Rohlmann A, Bergmann G. Influence of different artificial disc kinematics on spine biomechanics. Clin Biomech Bristol Avon febrero de 2009; 24(2): 135-42.
[http://dx.doi.org/10.1016/j.clinbiomech.2008.11.008]

[101] Kim HS, Wu PH, Jang IT. Lumbar Degenerative disease part 1: anatomy and pathophysiology of intervertebral discogenic pain and radiofrequency ablation of basivertebral and sinuvertebral nerve treatment for chronic discogenic back pain: a prospective case series and review of literature. Int J Mol Sci 2020; 21(4): 1483.
[http://dx.doi.org/10.3390/ijms21041483] [PMID: 32098249]

[102] Centeno C, Markle J, Dodson E, *et al.* Treatment of lumbar degenerative disc disease-associated radicular pain with culture-expanded autologous mesenchymal stem cells: a pilot study on safety and efficacy. J Transl Med 2017; 15(1): 197.
[http://dx.doi.org/10.1186/s12967-017-1300-y] [PMID: 28938891]

[103] Zheng J, Shen C. [Retracted] quantitative relationship between the degree of lumbar disc degeneration and intervertebral disc height in patients with low back pain. Contrast Media Mol Imaging 2022; 2022(1): 5960317.
[http://dx.doi.org/10.1155/2022/5960317] [PMID: 35935310]

[104] Beatty S. We need to talk about lumbar total disc replacement. Int J Spine Surg 2018; 12(2): 201-40.
[http://dx.doi.org/10.14444/5029] [PMID: 30276080]

[105] Othman YA, Verma R, Qureshi SA. Artificial disc replacement in spine surgery. Ann Transl Med 2019; 7(S5) (Suppl. 5): S170.
[http://dx.doi.org/10.21037/atm.2019.08.26] [PMID: 31624736]

[106] Modic MT. Degenerative disc disease: genotyping, MR imaging and phenotyping. Skeletal Radiol 2006; 36(2): 91-3.
[http://dx.doi.org/10.1007/s00256-006-0159-4] [PMID: 16738912]

[107] Modic MT, Steinberg PM, Ross JS, Masaryk TJ, Carter JR. Degenerative disk disease: assessment of changes in vertebral body marrow with MR imaging. Radiology 1988; 166(1): 193-9.
[http://dx.doi.org/10.1148/radiology.166.1.3336678] [PMID: 3336678]

[108] Fujiwara A, Tamai K, Yamato M, *et al.* The relationship between facet joint osteoarthritis and disc degeneration of the lumbar spine: an MRI study. Eur Spine J 1999; 8(5): 396-401.
[http://dx.doi.org/10.1007/s005860050193] [PMID: 10552323]

[109] Pathria M, Sartoris DJ, Resnick D. Osteoarthritis of the facet joints: accuracy of oblique radiographic assessment. Radiology 1987; 164(1): 227-30.
[http://dx.doi.org/10.1148/radiology.164.1.3588910] [PMID: 3588910]

[110] Rohlmann A, Lauterborn S, Dreischarf M, *et al.* Parameters influencing the outcome after total disc replacement at the lumbosacral junction. Part 1: misalignment of the vertebrae adjacent to a total disc replacement affects the facet joint and facet capsule forces in a probabilistic finite element analysis. Eur Spine J 2013; 22(10): 2271-8.
[http://dx.doi.org/10.1007/s00586-013-2909-z] [PMID: 23868223]

[111] Takigawa T, Espinoza Orías AA, An HS, *et al.* Spinal kinematics and facet load transmission after total disc replacement. Spine 2010; 35(22): E1160-6.
[http://dx.doi.org/10.1097/BRS.0b013e3181e5352d] [PMID: 20881657]

[112] Le Huec JC, Lafage V, Bonnet X, *et al.* Validated finite element analysis of the maverick total disc prosthesis. J Spinal Disord Tech 2010; 23(4): 249-57.
[http://dx.doi.org/10.1097/BSD.0b013e3181a5db24] [PMID: 20068471]

[113] Hitchon PW, Eichholz K, Barry C, *et al.* Biomechanical studies of an artificial disc implant in the human cadaveric spine. J Neurosurg Spine 2005; 2(3): 339-43.
[http://dx.doi.org/10.3171/spi.2005.2.3.0339] [PMID: 15796360]

[114] Dreischarf M, Schmidt H, Putzier M, Zander T. Biomechanics of the L5–S1 motion segment after total disc replacement – Influence of iatrogenic distraction, implant positioning and preoperative disc height on the range of motion and loading of facet joints. J Biomech 2015; 48(12): 3283-91.
[http://dx.doi.org/10.1016/j.jbiomech.2015.06.023] [PMID: 26184587]

[115] Kim SW, Paik SH, Oh JK, Kwak YH, Lee HW, You KH. The impact of coronal alignment of device on radiographic degeneration in the case of total disc replacement. Spine J 2016; 16(4): 470-9.
[http://dx.doi.org/10.1016/j.spinee.2015.07.436] [PMID: 26208879]

[116] Serhan H, Mhatre D, Defossez H, Bono CM. Motion-preserving technologies for degenerative lumbar spine: The past, present, and future horizons. SAS J 2011; 5(3): 75-89.
[http://dx.doi.org/10.1016/j.esas.2011.05.001] [PMID: 25802672]

[117] Enker P, Steffee A, Mcmillin C, Keppler L, Biscup R, Miller S. Artificial disc replacement. Preliminary report with a 3-year minimum follow-up. Spine 1993; 18(8): 1061-70.
[http://dx.doi.org/10.1097/00007632-199306150-00017] [PMID: 8367774]

[118] Devin CJ, Myers TG, Kang JD. Chronic failure of a lumbar total disc replacement with osteolysis. Report of a case with nineteen-year follow-up. J Bone Joint Surg Am 2008; 90(10): 2230-4.
[http://dx.doi.org/10.2106/JBJS.G.01712] [PMID: 18829921]

[119] Schmidt H, Midderhoff S, Adkins K, Wilke HJ. The effect of different design concepts in lumbar total disc arthroplasty on the range of motion, facet joint forces and instantaneous center of rotation of a L4-5 segment. Eur Spine J 2009; 18(11): 1695-705.
[http://dx.doi.org/10.1007/s00586-009-1146-y] [PMID: 19763638]

[120] Kostuik JP. Complications and surgical revision for failed disc arthroplasty. Spine J 2004; 4(6) (Suppl.): S289-91.
[http://dx.doi.org/10.1016/j.spinee.2004.07.021] [PMID: 15541678]

[121] Gamradt SC, Wang JC. Lumbar disc arthroplasty. Spine J 2005; 5(1): 95-103.
[http://dx.doi.org/10.1016/j.spinee.2004.09.006] [PMID: 15653090]

[122] Kurtz SM, Peloza J, Siskey R, Villarraga ML. Analysis of a retrieved polyethylene total disc replacement component. Spine J 2005; 5(3): 344-50.
[http://dx.doi.org/10.1016/j.spinee.2004.11.011] [PMID: 15863092]

[123] Rousseau MA, Bradford DS, Bertagnoli R, Hu SS, Lotz JC. Disc arthroplasty design influences intervertebral kinematics and facet forces. Spine J 2006; 6(3): 258-66.
[http://dx.doi.org/10.1016/j.spinee.2005.07.004] [PMID: 16651219]

[124] Punt IM, Visser VM, van Rhijn LW, *et al.* Complications and reoperations of the SB Charité lumbar disc prosthesis: experience in 75 patients. Eur Spine J 2008; 17(1): 36-43.
[http://dx.doi.org/10.1007/s00586-007-0506-8] [PMID: 17929065]

[125] Shim CS, Lee SH, Shin HD, *et al.* CHARITE *versus* ProDisc: a comparative study of a minimum 3-year follow-up. Spine 2007; 32(9): 1012-8.
[http://dx.doi.org/10.1097/01.brs.0000260795.57798.a0] [PMID: 17450077]

[126] Siepe CJ, Korge A, Grochulla F, Mehren C, Mayer HM. Analysis of post-operative pain patterns following total lumbar disc replacement: results from fluoroscopically guided spine infiltrations. Eur Spine J 2008; 17(1): 44-56.
[http://dx.doi.org/10.1007/s00586-007-0519-3] [PMID: 17972116]

[127] Punt I, van Rijsbergen M, van Rietbergen B, *et al.* Subsidence of SB Charité total disc replacement and the role of undersizing. Eur Spine J 2013; 22(10): 2264-70.
[http://dx.doi.org/10.1007/s00586-013-2864-8] [PMID: 23771503]

[128] Kurtz SM, van Ooij A, Ross R, *et al.* Polyethylene wear and rim fracture in total disc arthroplasty. Spine J 2007; 7(1): 12-21.
[http://dx.doi.org/10.1016/j.spinee.2006.05.012] [PMID: 17197327]

[129] Mayer HM. Total lumbar disc replacement. J Bone Joint Surg Br agosto de 2005; 87(8): 1029-37.

[130] Ross R, Mirza AH, Norris HE, Khatri M. Survival and clinical outcome of SB Charité III disc replacement for back pain. J Bone Joint Surg Br 2007; 89-B(6): 785-9.
[http://dx.doi.org/10.1302/0301-620X.89B6.18806] [PMID: 17613505]

[131] Gragnaniello C, Seex KA, Eisermann LG, Claydon MH, Malham GM. Early postoperative dislocation of the anterior Maverick lumbar disc prosthesis. J Neurosurg Spine 2013; 19(2): 191-6.
[http://dx.doi.org/10.3171/2013.5.SPINE12753] [PMID: 23768025]

[132] Eliasberg CD, Kelly MP, Ajiboye RM, SooHoo NF. Complications and rates of subsequent lumbar surgery following lumbar total disc arthroplasty and lumbar fusion. Spine 2016; 41(2): 173-81.
[http://dx.doi.org/10.1097/BRS.0000000000001180] [PMID: 26751061]

[133] Sasso RC, Foulk DM, Hahn M. Prospective, randomized trial of metal-on-metal artificial lumbar disc replacement: initial results for treatment of discogenic pain. Spine 2008; 33(2): 123-31.
[http://dx.doi.org/10.1097/BRS.0b013e31816043af] [PMID: 18197095]

[134] Valdevit A, Errico TJ. Design and evaluation of the FlexiCore metal-on-metal intervertebral disc prosthesis. Spine J 2004; 4(6) (Suppl.): S276-88.
[http://dx.doi.org/10.1016/j.spinee.2004.07.016] [PMID: 15541677]

[135] Cinotti G, David T, Postacchini F. Results of disc prosthesis after a minimum follow-up period of 2 years. Spine 1996; 21(8): 995-1000.
[http://dx.doi.org/10.1097/00007632-199604150-00015] [PMID: 8726204]

[136] Griffith SL, Shelokov AP, Büttner-Janz K, LeMaire JP, Zeegers WS. A multicenter retrospective study of the clinical results of the LINK SB Charité intervertebral prosthesis. The initial European experience. Spine 1994; 19(16): 1842-9.
[http://dx.doi.org/10.1097/00007632-199408150-00009] [PMID: 7973983]

[137] Lee CK, Goel VK. Artificial disc prosthesis: design concepts and criteria. Spine J 2004; 4(6) (Suppl.): S209-18.
[http://dx.doi.org/10.1016/j.spinee.2004.07.011] [PMID: 15541669]

[138] Eskander MS, Onyedika II, Eskander JP, Connolly PJ, Eck JC, Lapinsky A. Revision strategy for posterior extrusion of the CHARITÉ polyethylene core. Spine 2010; 35(24): E1430-4.
[http://dx.doi.org/10.1097/BRS.0b013e3181e9bf30] [PMID: 21030890]

[139] Jeon SH, Choi WG, Lee SH. Anterior revision of a dislocated ProDisc prosthesis at the L4-5 level. J Spinal Disord Tech 2008; 21(6): 448-50.
[http://dx.doi.org/10.1097/BSD.0b013e3181633a32] [PMID: 18679102]

[140] Baxter RM, MacDonald DW, Kurtz SM, Steinbeck MJ. Severe impingement of lumbar disc replacements increases the functional biological activity of polyethylene wear debris. J Bone Joint Surg Am 2013; 95(11): e75.
[http://dx.doi.org/10.2106/JBJS.K.00522] [PMID: 23780545]

[141] Zeegers WS, Bohnen LMLJ, Laaper M, Verhaegen MJA. Artificial disc replacement with the modular type SB Charité III: 2-year results in 50 prospectively studied patients. Eur Spine J 1999; 8(3): 210-7.
[http://dx.doi.org/10.1007/s005860050160] [PMID: 10413347]

[142] van Ooij A, Kurtz SM, Stessels F, Noten H, van Rhijn L. Polyethylene wear debris and long-term clinical failure of the Charité disc prosthesis: a study of 4 patients. Spine 2007; 32(2): 223-9.
[PMID: 17224818]

[143] Fraser RD, Ross ER, Lowery GL, Freeman BJ, Dolan M. AcroFlex design and results. Spine J 2004; 4(6) (Suppl.): S245-51.
[http://dx.doi.org/10.1016/j.spinee.2004.07.020] [PMID: 15541673]

[144] Veruva SY, Lanman TH, Isaza JE, Freeman TA, Kurtz SM, Steinbeck MJ. Periprosthetic UHMWPE wear debris induces inflammation, vascularization, and innervation after total disc replacement in the lumbar spine. Clin Orthop Relat Res 2017; 475(5): 1369-81.
[PMID: 27488379]

[145] Wright TM. CORR insights®: Periprosthetic UHMWPE wear debris induces inflammation, vascularization, and innervation after total disc replacement in the lumbar spine. Clin Orthop Relat Res 2017; 475(5): 1382-5.
[PMID: 27535283]

[146] Werner JH, Rosenberg JH, Keeley KL, Agrawal DK. Immunobiology of periprosthetic inflammation and pain following ultra-high-molecular-weight-polyethylene wear debris in the lumbar spine. Expert Rev Clin Immunol 2018; 14(8): 695-706.
[PMID: 30099915]

[147] Berry MR, Peterson BG, Alander DH. A granulomatous mass surrounding a Maverick total disc replacement causing iliac vein occlusion and spinal stenosis: a case report. J Bone Joint Surg Am 2010; 92(5): 1242-5.
[PMID: 20439671]

[148] François J, Coessens R, Lauweryns P. Early removal of a Maverick disc prosthesis: surgical findings and morphological changes. Acta Orthop Belg 2007; 73(1): 122-7.
[PMID: 17441671]

[149] David T. Lumbar disc prosthesis. Surgical technique, indications and clinical results in 22 patients with a minimum of 12 months follow-up. Eur Spine J 1993; 1(4): 254-9.
[PMID: 20054928]

[150] Tropiano P, Huang RC, Girardi FP, Cammisa FP Jr, Marnay T. Lumbar total disc replacement. Surgical technique. J Bone Joint Surg Am 2006; 88 (Suppl. 1 Pt 1): 50-64.
[PMID: 16510800]

[151] Geisler FH. Surgical technique of lumbar artificial disc replacement with the Charité artificial disc. Neurosurgery 2005; 56(1) (Suppl.): 46-57.
[PMID: 15799792]

[152] Sharabi M, Levi-Sasson A, Wolfson R, Wade KR, Galbusera F, Benayahu D, *et al.* The mechanical role of the radial fibers network within the annulus fibrosus of the lumbar intervertebral disc: a finite elements study. J Biomech Eng 2018.
[PMID: 30758511]

[153] Cakir B, Schmidt R, Mattes T, Fraitzl CR, Reichel H, Käfer W. Index level mobility after total lumbar disc replacement: is it beneficial or detrimental? Spine 2009; 34(9): 917-23.
[PMID: 19532000]

[154] Mobbs RJ, Li JXJ, Phan K. Anterior longitudinal ligament reconstruction to reduce hypermobility of cervical and lumbar disc arthroplasty. Asian Spine J 2017; 11(6): 943-50.
[PMID: 29279750]

[155] Tavakoli J, Diwan AD, Tipper JL. Advanced strategies for the regeneration of lumbar disc annulus fibrosus. Int J Mol Sci 2020; 21(14): 4889.
[PMID: 32664453]

CHAPTER 3

Lumbar Interbody Fusion: Different Approaches and Biomechanical Issues

Máximo Alberto Díez-Ulloa[1,*], Luis Puente-Sánchez[1] and Eva Díez-Sanchidrián[2]

[1] *Spinal Unit, Orthopedics Department, University Hospital Complex of Santiago de Compostela, Santiago de Compostela, Spain*

[2] *Faculty of Medicine, University of Santiago de Compostela, Santiago de Compostela, Spain*

Abstract: Fusion is frequently considered when planning for a spinal surgery procedure; nowadays, such a fusion is preferred between the intervertebral bodies (so-called *interbody fusion*) because there is a bigger surface for the bone to grow and make contact (increasing fusion rates), improving also overall spine alignment (trying to get a balanced spine), which in turn protects the adjacent segment, as there is also less wobbling at the fused space and mechanic aspects are less deleterious.

From a mechanical point of view, a fusion is an ankylosing procedure that eliminates any movement between vertebral bodies, so the Functional Spine Unit (FSU) is abolished; both kinetics (forces at stake), kinematics (displacements caused by those forces) and stiffness (deformations by those same forces) within FSU should be considered.

Keywords: ALIF, Lumbar interbody fusion, OLIF, PLIF, TLIF, XLIF.

INTRODUCTION

Nowadays, a fusion of vertebral bodies is one of the most common surgical procedures performed worldwide. It implies bridging the selected vertebrae with bone tissue without a gap between them. Anatomically, that bridge may form in the posterior elements (laminae, facets, transverse apophyses) or in between the endplates of vertebral bodies: it is in this situation that we talk about interbody fusion, packing bone in the intervertebral disc space after removing the cartilaginous endplates. Some annulus fibrosus is kept in place as a safety measure to avoid either over distraction or intracanal migration of the graft or implants placed. It is important to highlight this point on graft, as fusion requires

---

* **Corresponding author Máximo Alberto Díez-Ulloa:** Spinal Unit, Orthopedics Department, University Hospital Complex of Santiago de Compostela, Santiago de Compostela, Spain; E-mail: maximoalberto.diez@usc.es

Javier Melchor Duart Clemente (Ed.)

bone tissue formation, not just an implant set between endplates to stabilize them (nevertheless, as any rule has exceptions, something that safely anchors to both endplates and incorporates into both vertebral bodies might pose such an exception), such as porous metallic blocks or cages.

So once established that we need to form a stable composite capable of withstanding physiological forces between vertebral bodies, two more issues should be addressed: a) how do we get there?; and b) how do we create a favorable environment for the bony bridge to grow, both from a mechanical and a biological viewpoint?

How do we Get there? The Surgical Approach

There are several acronyms regarding interbody approach fusion. To ease understanding, a root, and a prefix may help the reader to understand this. The root word is -LIF, which stands for *Lumbar Interbody Fusion* (LIF). We may extend the L to the Thoracic spine, with two core differences: a) the rib cage and the thoracic cavity, which makes the thoracic spine less mobile than the lumbar spine, and b) the anterior approaches have to deal with the pleural cavities, which are physiologically different to the peritoneum; for instance, they have a negative pressure during inspiration, suctioning every loose matter (this can be avoided access the spine through a retropleural approach). The cervical spine has considerations that go way beyond this chapter.

Let us think about a transverse anatomical slice at the level of a lumbar disc in a supine patient, the standard CT or MRI axial cuts. If we go around the clock, then we have several approaches: a)ALIF (anterior, straight from the front, at 12:00, either -mostly- retroperitoneal or else transperitoneal), b)OLIF (oblique) between the great vessels and the psoas, c)XLIF (*extreme lateral*) through the psoas -by splitting fibers, at 3:00-: d)TLIF (*transforaminal*, approximately at 5:00), through the foramen, but lateral to the dural sac (with its variation e-TLIF, extreme-transforaminal, from the back but quite lateral from the facets); and e)PLIF (posterior, at 6:00), retracting the dural sac to the midline to create the approach.

They all have pros and cons, and some anatomical specificities make the surgeon choose one over another when planning a LIF technique. The anatomy of the great vessels and the nerve roots have a bearing on the anterior approaches: while on the one hand, the L5-S1 level is easily accessible through ALIF, the L4-L5 level is the big puzzle, as the aortic and iliac bifurcations usually lie there, with a gross lumbar vein tying the great vessels (making it almost mandatory to ligate it in case mobilization is needed). The psoas has up to 80% of the cross-sectional area with a nerve root in the way of a direct lateral approach -the percentage of which progressively decreases at the more cranial levels-; thus the Oblique

(OLIF) might be a choice if the vascular anatomy allows for it (there must be a corridor between the great vessels and the psoas muscle). On the downside of the OLIF, the interbody implant insertion needs a rotation of 30° that the iliac crest may hamper. Among the posterior approaches, the TLIF leaves the dural sac untouched and protected by the ligamentum flavum, and the sac needs no retraction.

Should an Implant be Placed in the Interbody Space?

Although increasing the overall cost and lengthening the surgical time, there are several reasons for this:

a) Higher Fusion Rate

Higher fusion rate anterior structural support adds stability. A recent meta-analysis confirms this assertion [1]. The optimal conditions for an interbody fusion (graft incorporation) are as follows:

1) Forces and stresses acting at the graft-host interface should not exceed its failure limits;

2) The stresses´ average (stress, by definition, being a load that causes a deformation) should not sum up to zero, because bone growth is enhanced by loads; and

3) Cyclic variations in stress are beneficial unless motion (mostly shear) occurs at the graft-host interface.

Historically, two models have been proposed [2]:

1) The tripod: anterior cancellous graft and posterior distraction.

2) The flagpole: anterior interbody distraction with a block and posterior compression.

Due to global spinal alignment reasons, only the second has stood the test of time; the tripod had built a flat back and imbalanced the spine.

b) Alignment of the Sagittal Plane

Alignment of the sagittal plane by increasing segmental lordosis, hence the importance of something structural to withstand axial forces at the intervertebral space until the bone bridges become strong enough by themselves at the anterior column and in the posterior one (in the midline, facets or intertransverse area).

The Lumbar lordosis is the key to both radiological and clinical success, in total amount and shape altogether. It can be obtained with ALIF, OLIF, and LLIF better than with TLIF or PLIF, which surprisingly achieve no significant lordosis (on average, around a 5° gain [3, 4]). Anyhow, if there is no anterior structural support, a void in the anterior column will bring about collapse and kyphosis.

c) Protection of the Adjacent Segment

The degenerated disc has irregular mechanics, and an implant increases stiffness. It is noteworthy that biomechanical properties of disc tissue bring about an erratic behavior of the instant center of rotation of the functional spine unit, something like a ramshackle crankshaft unsteadily rotating. This situation results in unpredictable behavior for a single patient and, mostly, irregular cycling with load spikes transferred to posterior implants. Nonetheless, some recent research shows that this is not as crucial as previously thought [5].

d) Damaged Tissue Removal

As the remaining disc tissue could potentially be a source of pain by itself, the more of it removed, the better.

e) Clinical Outcome

Long-term follow-up research supports a better outcome for patients with circumferential *versus* posterolateral lumbar fusion [6, 7].

What are the Arguments against this Need?

Recent literature states that there is no clear-cut difference in clinical outcomes in degenerative spondylolisthesis patients, but some key aspects show improvement with LIF regarding both fusion rates and alignment among other advantages [8], as well as some protective effects for early screw loosening [9]. Others disregard the extra cost of LIF in patients operated on for degenerative spondylolisthesis, with similar costs and outcomes, but with older age in PLF *vs.* TLIF patients [10].

Another issue to consider is the risk of subsidence (collapse into subchondral bone, therefore endangering the anterior support which could eventually be lost), especially if too big and rigid implants without any load transfer to the circumferential cortices, particularly in osteoporotic bone. Subsidence is a topic for research on design and materials for interbody fusion implants, way beyond this chapter.

How do we Create a Favorable Environment?

To dig into the environment for interbody fusion, biomechanics need to be understood. It is the cornerstone of this chapter in this book. As clinicians, biomechanics is usually an intricate matter, so there is a need to introduce some explanation.

Guide of Biomechanics for Spine Doctors

Mathematics rules out anything about Mechanics, so the language needs to be precise and rationally based, with no room for interpretation. Because of this high level of certainty, we need assumptions to make Mathematics work with full power in the real world, but we will come back to this issue in this chapter.

We have focused on the Mechanics of the spine to understand what is at stake when we perform an interbody fusion from a purely physical point of view. To this, we add Biology, and then we have an almost complete picture of interbody fusion (almost, to leave something to that weird factor that makes things go not in an ideal way exactly).

The first thing to consider is the unit we work with: the Functional Spine Unit (FSU), composed of two adjacent vertebrae plus the facets, ligaments, and the disc between them. Then, whenever a force acts on a body, this body either moves (transforms such energy into kinetic energy) or else deforms (changes its shape), and probably always there is a mixture of the two. But for a better understanding, we will disregard deformation for this chapter; when deformation is the most important over motion, we deal with fractures.

We need to know that we approach Mechanics from two perspectives: kinetics and kinematics. Kinetics studies the forces within the element (the FSU) and absolute motion (static or dynamic), focusing on the action of forces producing or changing such a motion. Whilst Kinematics studies the displacements, the position of this element referenced to others, the relative motion. So, this is the Mechanics of motion without reference to the forces causing it. The variables are position, acceleration, and velocity.

Let's remember some engineering definitions:

a. An element is any of the unitary mechanical parts used for building blocks in the design of machines;
b. A body is a collection of matter analyzed as a single object;
c. A rigid body is a collection of particles with the property that the distances between particles remain unchanged during the course of motions of the body;

and

d. A composite is the macroscopic combination of two or more distinct materials with a definite interface between them.

In aN FSU, the vertebral bodies remain rigid (assumption: we disregard the possible deformation inside it), while the disc is a deformable body that allows for motion between vertebral bodies, and the FSU is a composite. With an interbody fusion, we intend to transform a FSU into one only body.

Research on Biomechanics can be made with specimens or with mathematical models, specifically Finite Element Models. The former is with some parts of the spine devoid of muscles and soft tissues around (with the exception, of course, of ligaments, discs, and facet capsules), which are then fixed at both ends, and loads are applied to measure displacements or *vice versa*; the specimen is soaked or submerged in saline to preserve tissue properties. The assumption is made on the absolute fixation at the ends, and assimilation of a live human spine to a cadaveric one (usually fresh frozen and then thawed under strict conditions), or else a porcine or bovine spine is performed. With the FEM, we recreate and design a model made of minute voxels to which we confer specific properties, afterward diverse load regimes are applied, and recording of what happens through several variables is done. A mathematical model needs assimilation into some mechanical model and tuning by specimens.

A beam is a structural element that primarily resists loads applied laterally (perpendicular to) regarding its axis and deforms by bending, with a different behavior whether fixation is on one side or both and whether the load is applied to the free end or somewhere (center or off-center) along it. This deformation is called deflection (it may be measured as a distance or as an angle). There are formulas to calculate such deflections: in the case of complex 3D bodies, a stiffness matrix seems the most appropriate. The stiffness matrix method (also known as the direct stiffness method) is particularly suitable for computerized analyses of statically indeterminate structures like the FSU (a statically indeterminate structure cannot be analyzed using only equilibrium equations). In this setting, the system must become a set of idealized elements interconnected at the nodes, the FSU as a beam with both vertebrae being two nodes, then the material stiffness properties (displacements, rotations) are compiled into a single matrix equation that determines unknown displacements or rotation when solved. This stiffness matrix is the basis for Finite Element Analysis studies.

A stiffness matrix is created based on three perpendicular axes and the relative motion of one point A about another point B (considered fixed) in all three planes (a plane defined by every two axes), including displacement and rotation (referenced to each axis) deflection of a beam defined by points A and B. It's assumed that the FSU has a beam-like behavior [11]. Point A in our scope is the center of the vertebra to which loads are applied, and point B is the center of the other vertebra, FSU being A plus B. There is a 6x6 matrix because the motion has 6 degrees of freedom: 3 for displacement and 3 for rotation; after all, there are three axes for coordinates. In frame structure, there are three forces: axial, shear, and rotational; or else, alongside, perpendicular to, or around each axis. Again, making some assumptions, we simplify it and divide it by a diagonal so that there are only 21 out of 36 data. Thus, we calculate the eventual displacements of A about B under varying conditions. Nonetheless, the descriptions of relative motion about a fixed point (the B vertebra) cannot comply with coupled motions, so the direct translation of results into clinics must be cautious.

We try to recreate the physiological environment with a wet environment for the specimen during the tests, and preload to assimilate to real-life conditions. A preload is a load placed on a body before any testing, and it needs some time to cause its full effect and some relaxation time for such an effect to disappear (and sometimes it does not disappear completely). Regarding this preload, we can find values from 300 to 500 N of axial compressive tension, and the applied flexion-extension moments 7.5-8 Nm (which are the assumptions for an accepted physiological environment in a human lumbar spine). Preloading (250 N for standing and 500 N for seating) increases the stiffness of the FSU. The 500 N preloading means stiffness 7x for lateral bending (X rotation in this case) and 3x for the lateral translation (X rotation and Y axis displacement, respectively [12].

We apply loads and measure the displacements (translations and rotations) and *viceversa* for each axis. Thence, we obtain hysteresis loops for each (in the plane perpendicular to each axis) which makes up six graphs, one for each degree of freedom. Hysteresis is the phenomenon in which the value of a physical property lags behind changes in the effect causing it to change (see Figs. 1 and 2). Let a load cause a displacement or rotation, and that load recedes, displacement or rotation comes back, but not at the same pace and not linearly. The load-displacement curve of an FSU shows a non-linear behavior in most dimensions, which means that the load causes a displacement, and when that load disappears, the return path is not the same: a loop is drawn instead of a straight line. This loop is called a hysteresis loop and is related to energy transfer and recovery.

Vertebral bodies of the FSU are assumed rigid, so deflection of the AB beam takes place in the disc, and such deflection is directly related to the mechanical properties of that disc. We know that when degenerated, the disc changes its properties causing the instant center of rotation to lose its usual displacement along FSU motion and become erratic, thus altering the properties of FSU.

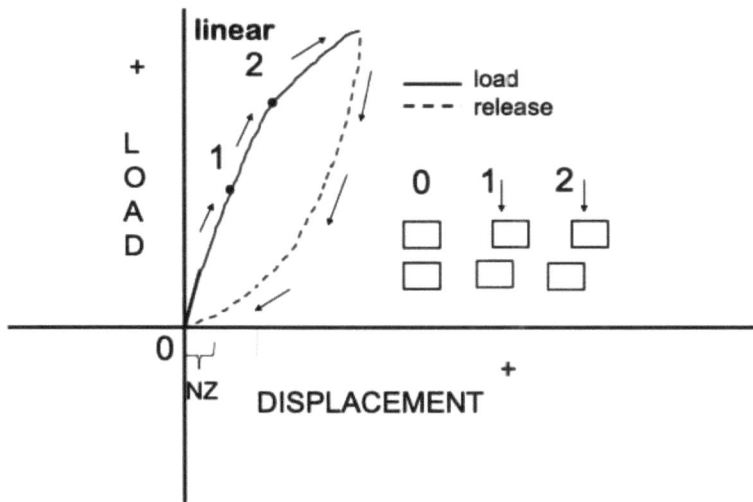

Fig. (1). Load-displacement curves, linear behavior: up and down in an almost straight line (Hysteresis loop). The area between the curves proportionally reflects energy loss.

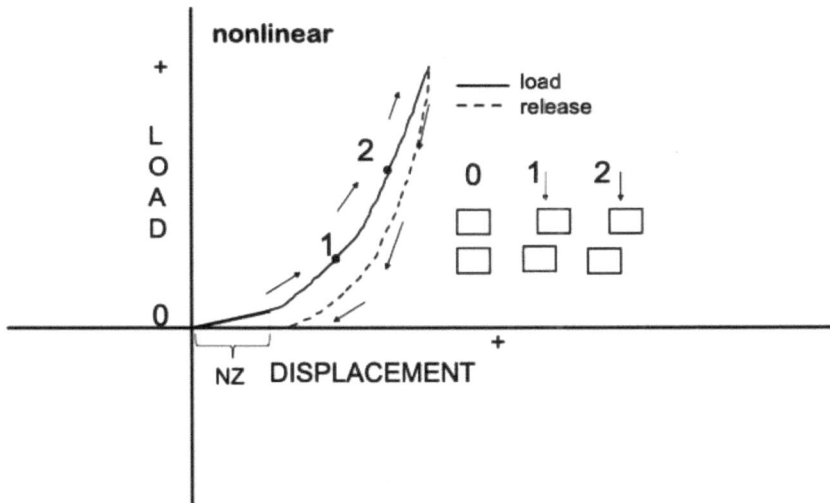

Fig. (2). Load-displacement curves, non-linear behavior: there is a zone (NZ: neutral zone) in which minimal forces cause displacement. Afterward, proportionally more load is needed to create the same displacement.

Test conditions are paramount to interpreting the results. Gardner defines displacements of + 0.5 mm in both AP and lateral directions, + 0,35 in the axial direction, + 1.5° lateral bending rotation and + 1° flexion-extension and torsional rotations, and assumed these data from a previous study on the physiological range of motion of FSU [13].

An important biomechanical concept is the Neutral Zone (NZ). In these hysteresis loops of the motion segment testing, there is a Neutral Zone (NZ), which (after Smit [14]) is the region of minimal stiffness or maximal compliance of a spinal motion segment (see Fig. 1). The NZ definition is a region of intervertebral motion around the neutral posture in which the passive spine offers little resistance [15]. The difference is not in the concept but in the way it is measured, either with angles (Panjabi) or through a mathematical model (Smit). This NZ changes with degenerative changes, an increase in the NZ might be a better indicator for degeneration or injury (that is, it moves with less energy transmission) than the ROM at a definite segment in biomechanical studies [16].

Another concept that deserves mention is the follower load, described in 1999 [17]; it is the path the load takes along the spine. If it is transferred tangent to the spine alignment (perpendicular to the end plates), then the load-carrying capacity of the spine is much higher than in a purely vertical axial mode on top (10x). In other words, loads are rerouted through the centers of gravity of vertebral bodies and impinge perpendicularly on the middle vertebral endplate and disc below. Without the stabilizing muscle action, the spine could not withstand a physiological load. With a follower preload as high as 1200N, up to 75% or 85% of ROM in flexion-extension is possible [18]. A follower load is a stabilization mechanism for the spine through muscle control [19] (see Fig. 3).

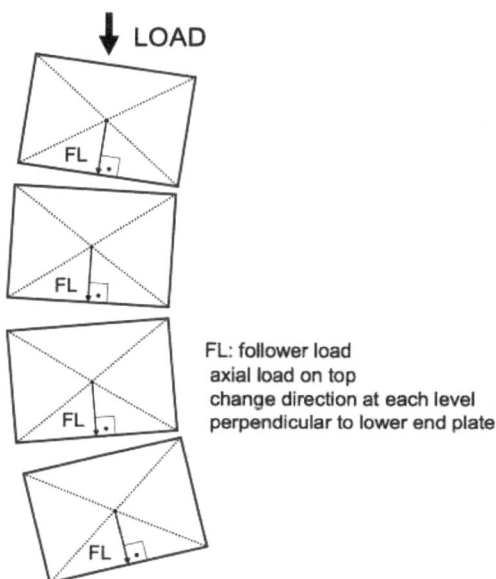

Fig. (3). Comparison of pure axial load *vs.* follower load; muscles create an FL scenario.

Testing a low-degeneration specimen for load-displacement curves after sequential injury of some structures (ligaments, facets, nucleus pulposus) showed some pre-tensioning as their injury changed lordosis at rest, and the most influential on segment stability was the nucleus pulposus [20]. An objective was to formulate transferable data for finite-element model calibration, which also showed the non-linear behavior of the FSU. However, the study consisted of the sequential sectioning of structures without addressing tissue interactions.

A look into the future: the to-do list (personal selection) [21].

• Develop stiffness matrices that reflect the non-linear behavior of the FSU.
• Account for aging effects in terms of disc degeneration.
• Connect *in vitro* FSU properties with *in vivo* observations.

FINAL REMARKS

Never forget that finite-element studies are not real-life, be cautious about interpretation and translation to clinics because of high inter-subject variability, and better use instead a pooled median of results of individual models [22]. When reading about Biomechanics as a surgeon, have a critical appraisal. Always check whether it is a specimen (human or other) or a finite-element model study. Then check the conditions and assumptions, for example, preload (yes or no) and how much, moments applied, model, *etc.* For example, see the linear effect of an increasing preload on intact spinal segments (0N, then 200 N, and then 400 N) [23]. Now you can read and drive to your own conclusions and compare with similar papers.

AND NOW FOR THE FSU-INTERBODY FUSION CLINICAL STUDIES

With all this in mind (take a few minutes to rest if you need to digest and assimilate all that information) it's easier to understand what we read, as surgeons, when dealing with biomechanical papers.

In a LIF testing experiment, we substitute the disc of the FSU with an implant under different conditions and measure the hysteresis loops, trying to find the minimal displacement possible (the most stable construct) for a LIF. If the reader is interested in a historical perspective of interbody fusion, read the paper by de Kunder [24].

Against some previous papers and assumptions, the approach is not the key for segmental or lumbar lordosis [25 - 28]: ALIF, LLIF, and TLIF get around 3.6° to 7°, differences, if any, being not noteworthy. In another study, OLIF showed around the same degree of correction (4.4°)². Even more interesting is that total lumbar lordosis changes are less significant than segmental lordosis. LLIF and PLIF constructs in a cadaveric model (L2-L5 segments, working on the L3-L4) had similar stabilizing effects, especially with a bilateral pedicle screw construct [29]. With MIS on the rise, there is a galore focus on new technical variants. Research on lateral MI approaches: ELIF plus unilateral pedicle screws plus transfacet screw behaved similarly to TLIF plus bilateral screws in a FEM model [30]; LLIF cages need posterior fixation in FEM [31].

Maybe the key is in the concept of restoration *vs.* creation. When there is an appropriate balance and anatomy preservation in the segment (high disc and low spinopelvic mismatch preoperatively), the gain in lordosis with a posterior cage will be less. But if the disc has shrunk, there is a vacuum sign, or the segment has collapsed, the increase in segmental lordosis will be higher [32]. In an all-*versus*-all LIF comparative literature review study [33], there was no difference among PLIF, TLIF, MI-TLIF, OLIF, LLIF, and ALIF in clinical outcomes and anterior support had a role in disc height restoration and sagittal contour. Also, PLF with no interbody fixation showed no differences in patient-reported outcomes (PROMs) in the short term. ALIF *vs.* TLIF systematic review and meta-analysis [34] showed similar fusion rates, neurological injuries, and infection rates, and ALIF had fewer dural injuries but more vessel injuries. PLIF *vs.* TLIF meta-analysis rendered no difference in outcomes, fusion, infection, or root injury, but PLIF had a higher complication rate [35].

CONCLUSION

• Critically appraise everything you read.

• Basic science management is a must.

• Interbody fusion helps fusion and alignment, although segmental lordosis is around 5°.

• Interbody fusion may protect screws from loosening.

• Posterior fixation adds stiffness to anterior devices.

REFERENCES

[1]   Dantas F, Dantas FLR, Botelho RV. Effect of interbody fusion compared with posterolateral fusion on lumbar degenerative spondylolisthesis: a systematic review and meta-analysis. Spine J 2022; 22(5): 756-68.
       [http://dx.doi.org/10.1016/j.spinee.2021.12.001] [PMID: 34896611]

[2]   Evans JH. Biomechanics of lumbar fusion. Clin Orthop Relat Res 1985; (193): 38-46.
       [PMID: 3882295]

[3]   Kepler CK, Rihn JA, Radcliff KE, *et al.* Restoration of lordosis and disk height after single-level

transforaminal lumbar interbody fusion. Orthop Surg 2012; 4(1): 15-20.
[http://dx.doi.org/10.1111/j.1757-7861.2011.00165.x] [PMID: 22290814]

[4] Rothrock RJ, McNeill IT, Yaeger K, Oermann EK, Cho SK, Caridi JM. Lumbar lordosis correction with interbody fusion. World Neurosurg 2018; 118: 21-31.
[http://dx.doi.org/10.1016/j.wneu.2018.06.216] [PMID: 29981462]

[5] Mesregah MK, Yoshida B, Lashkari N, *et al.* Demographic, clinical, and operative risk factors associated with postoperative adjacent segment disease in patients undergoing lumbar spine fusions: a systematic review and meta-analysis. Spine J 2022; 22(6): 1038-69.
[http://dx.doi.org/10.1016/j.spinee.2021.12.002] [PMID: 34896610]

[6] Videbaek TS, Christensen FB, Soegaard R, *et al.* Circumferential fusion improves outcome in comparison with instrumented posterolateral fusion: long-term results of a randomized clinical trial. Spine 2006; 31(25): 2875-80.
[http://dx.doi.org/10.1097/01.brs.0000247793.99827.b7] [PMID: 17139217]

[7] Soegaard R, Bünger CE, Christiansen T, Høy K, Eiskjaer SP, Christensen FB. Circumferential fusion is dominant over posterolateral fusion in a long-term perspective: cost-utility evaluation of a randomized controlled trial in severe, chronic low back pain. Spine 2007; 32(22): 2405-14.
[http://dx.doi.org/10.1097/BRS.0b013e3181573b2d] [PMID: 18090078]

[8] Carreon LY, Glassman S, Ghogawala Z, Mummaneni P. McGirt M, Asher A. Modeled cost-effectiveness of transforaminal lumbar interbody fusion for spondylolisthesis using N2QOD data. J Neurosurg Spine 2016; 24: 916-21.
[http://dx.doi.org/10.3171/2015.10.SPINE15917] [PMID: 26895529]

[9] Kim DH, Hwang RW, Lee GH, *et al.* Comparing rates of early pedicle screw loosening in posterolateral lumbar fusion with and without transforaminal lumbar interbody fusion. Spine J 2020; 20(9): 1438-45.
[http://dx.doi.org/10.1016/j.spinee.2020.04.021] [PMID: 32387295]

[10] Kim E, Chotai S, Stonko D, Wick J, Sielatycki A, Devin CJ. A retrospective review comparing two-year patient-reported outcomes, costs, and healthcare resource utilization for TLIF *vs.* PLF for single-level degenerative spondylolisthesis. Eur Spine J 2018; 27(3): 661-9.
[http://dx.doi.org/10.1007/s00586-017-5142-3] [PMID: 28585094]

[11] Gardner-Morse MG, Stokes IAF. Structural behavior of human lumbar spinal motion segments. J Biomech 2004; 37(2): 205-12.
[http://dx.doi.org/10.1016/j.jbiomech.2003.10.003] [PMID: 14706323]

[12] Stokes IA, Gardner-Morse M, Churchill D, Laible JP. Measurement of a spinal motion segment stiffness matrix. J Biomech 2002; 35(4): 517-21.
[http://dx.doi.org/10.1016/S0021-9290(01)00221-4] [PMID: 11934421]

[13] Marras WS, Lavender SA, Leurgans S, *et al.* Biomechanical risk factors for occupationally related low back disorders. Ergonomics 1995; 38(2): 377-410.
[http://dx.doi.org/10.1080/00140139508925111] [PMID: 7895740]

[14] Smit TH, van Tunen MSLM, van der Veen AJ, Kingma I, van Dieën JH. Quantifying intervertebral disc mechanics: a new definition of the neutral zone. BMC Musculoskelet Disord 2011; 12(1): 38-47.
[http://dx.doi.org/10.1186/1471-2474-12-38] [PMID: 21299900]

[15] Panjabi MM. The stabilizing system of the spine. Part II. Neutral zone and instability hypothesis. J Spinal Disord 1992; 5(4): 390-7.
[http://dx.doi.org/10.1097/00002517-199212000-00002] [PMID: 1490035]

[16] Panjabi M, Abumi K, Duranceau J, Oxland T. Spinal stability and intersegmental muscle forces. A biomechanical model. Spine 1989; 14(2): 194-200.
[http://dx.doi.org/10.1097/00007632-198902000-00008] [PMID: 2922640]

[17] Patwardhan AG, Havey RM, Meade KP, Lee B, Dunlap B. A follower load increases the load-carrying

capacity of the lumbar spine in compression. Spine 1999; 24(10): 1003-9.
[http://dx.doi.org/10.1097/00007632-199905150-00014] [PMID: 10332793]

[18]   Patwardhan AG, Havey RM, Carandang G, *et al.* Effect of compressive follower preload on the flexion–extension response of the human lumbar spine. J Orthop Res 2003; 21(3): 540-6.
[http://dx.doi.org/10.1016/S0736-0266(02)00202-4] [PMID: 12706029]

[19]   Kim B. A follower load as a muscle control mechanism to stabilize the lumbar spine 2011.
[http://dx.doi.org/10.17077/etd.4liqj2c0]

[20]   Heuer F, Schmidt H, Klezl Z, Claes L, Wilke HJ. Stepwise reduction of functional spinal structures increase range of motion and change lordosis angle. J Biomech 2007; 40(2): 271-80.
[http://dx.doi.org/10.1016/j.jbiomech.2006.01.007] [PMID: 16524582]

[21]   Oxland TR. Fundamental biomechanics of the spine—What we have learned in the past 25 years and future directions. J Biomech 2016; 49(6): 817-32.
[http://dx.doi.org/10.1016/j.jbiomech.2015.10.035] [PMID: 26706717]

[22]   Dreischarf M, Zander T, Shirazi-Adl A, *et al.* Comparison of eight published static finite element models of the intact lumbar spine: Predictive power of models improves when combined together. J Biomech 2014; 47(8): 1757-66.
[http://dx.doi.org/10.1016/j.jbiomech.2014.04.002] [PMID: 24767702]

[23]   Gardner-Morse MG, Stokes IA. Physiological axial compressive preloads increase motion segment stiffness, linearity and hysteresis in all six degrees of freedom for small displacements about the neutral posture. J Orthop Res 2003; 21(3): 547-52.
[http://dx.doi.org/10.1016/S0736-0266(02)00199-7] [PMID: 12706030]

[24]   de Kunder SL, Rijkers K, Caelers IJMH, de Bie RA, Koehler PJ, van Santbrink H. Lumbar interbody fusio. A historical overview and a future perspective. Spine 2018; 43(16): 1161-8.
[http://dx.doi.org/10.1097/BRS.0000000000002534] [PMID: 29280929]

[25]   Champagne PO, Walsh C, Diabira J, *et al.* Sagittal balance correction following lumbar interbody fusion: a comparison of three approaches. Asian Spine J 2019; 13(3): 450-8.
[http://dx.doi.org/10.31616/asj.2018.0128] [PMID: 30909679]

[26]   Martin CT, Niu S, Whicker E, Ward L, Yoon ST. Radiographic factors affecting lordosis correction after transforaminal lumbar interbody fusion with unilateral facetectomy. Int J Spine Surg 2020; 14(5): 681-6.
[http://dx.doi.org/10.14444/7099] [PMID: 33097580]

[27]   Berlin C, Zang F, Halm H, Quante M. Preoperative lordosis in L4/5 predicts segmental lordosis correction achievable by transforaminal lumbar interbody fusion. Eur Spine J 2021; 30(5): 1277-84.
[http://dx.doi.org/10.1007/s00586-020-06710-2] [PMID: 33409727]

[28]   Porche K, Dru A, Moor R, Kubilis P, Vaziri S, Hoh DJ. Preoperative radiographic prediction tool for early postoperative segmental and lumbar lordosis alignment after transforaminal lumbar interbody fusion. Cureus 2021; 13(9): e18175.
[http://dx.doi.org/10.7759/cureus.18175] [PMID: 34703700]

[29]   Godzik J, Kalb S, Reis M, *et al.* Biomechanical evaluation on interbody fixation with secondary augmentation: lateral lumbar interbody fusion versus posterior lumbar interbody fusion. 2018; 4: 180-6.
[http://dx.doi.org/10.21037/jss.2018.05.07]

[30]   Yang M, Sun G, Guo S, *et al.* The biomechanical study of extraforaminal lumbar interbody fusion: a three-dimensional finite-element analysis
[http://dx.doi.org/10.1155/2017/9365068]

[31]   Liu X, Ma J, Park P, Huang X, Xie N, Ye X. Biomechanical comparison of multilevel lateral interbody fusion with and without supplementary instrumentation: a three-dimensional finite element study. BMC Musculoskelet Disord 2017; 18(1): 63.

[http://dx.doi.org/10.1186/s12891-017-1387-6] [PMID: 28153036]

[32] Watkins RG IV, Hanna R, Chang D, Watkins RG III. Sagittal alignment after lumbar interbody fusion: comparing anterior, lateral, and transforaminal approaches. J Spinal Disord Tech 2014; 27(5): 253-6.
[http://dx.doi.org/10.1097/BSD.0b013e31828a8447] [PMID: 23511641]

[33] Divi SN, Schroeder GD, Goyal DKC, *et al.* Fusion technique does not affect short-term patient-reported outcomes for lumbar degenerative disease. Spine J 2019; 19(12): 1960-8.
[http://dx.doi.org/10.1016/j.spinee.2019.07.014] [PMID: 31355987]

[34] Phan K, Thayaparan GK, Mobbs RJ. Anterior lumbar interbody fusion *versus* transforaminal lumbar interbody fusion – systematic review and meta-analysis. Br J Neurosurg 2015; 29(5): 705-11.
[http://dx.doi.org/10.3109/02688697.2015.1036838] [PMID: 25968330]

[35] Zhang Q, Yuan Z, Zhou M, Liu H, Xu Y, Ren Y. A comparison of posterior lumbar interbody fusion and transforaminal lumbar interbody fusion: a literature review and meta-analysis. BMC Musculoskelet Disord 2014; 15(1): 367.
[http://dx.doi.org/10.1186/1471-2474-15-367] [PMID: 25373605]

CHAPTER 4

Management of Degenerative Spinal Conditions with Osteoporosis

Javier Cuarental García[1,*], **Luis Álvarez-Galovich**[1], **Félix Tomé-Bermejo**[1] and **Javier Melchor Duart-Clemente**[2]

[1] *Spinal Unit, FJD, Madrid, Spain*

[2] *Neurosurgery and Spinal Surgery Departments, Valencia General Hospital, Valencia, Spain*

Abstract: Osteoporosis is the most frequent metabolic bone disease, affecting particularly women. Due to the progressive ageing of the population, the number of patients with this condition requiring spine surgery is increasing, while new techniques and implants are in development to help this particular population: apart from percutaneous augmentation techniques (such as vertebroplasty and kyphoplasty), fenestrated pedicle screws which can be cemented have changed the spinal management of these patients.

Keywords: Bone cement, Degenerative spine, Fenestrated screws, Osteoporosis.

INTRODUCTION

Osteoporosis is the most frequent metabolic bone disease, which is characterized by a decrease in bone mass, a rate of bone resorption greater than synthesis, and microarchitectural deterioration [1]. This entails a decrease in the mechanical resistance of the bone and bone fragility and, consequently, an increased risk of fracture. Therefore, it is both a quantitative and qualitative alteration of the bone tissue.

The diagnosis is based on densitometry (DEXA) score: normal (T-score > -1 SD), osteopenia (T-score between -1 and -2,5 SD), and osteoporosis (T-score < -2,5 SD).

Epidemiology

This disease affects around 6% of men and 21% of women between the ages of 50 and 84 years in Europe n the European Union, around 27 million people

** Corresponding author Javier Cuarental García:** Spinal Unit, FJD, Madrid, Spain;
E-mail: javi_cuarental@hotmail.com

Javier Melchor Duart Clemente (Ed.)
All rights reserved-© 2025 Bentham Science Publishers

currently suffer from osteoporosis. It is estimated that in the next 10 years, the cases of this disease will increase by 23% [2].

It is estimated that 1 in 3 women over the age of 50 experience an osteoporosis-related fracture. Men have a lower risk of osteoporotic fracture but nevertheless, it is not trivial, reaching the maximum risk 10 years after women. Apart from age and gender, there are other risks factors, which can be found in Table **1**.

Table 1. Osteoporosis risks factors (modifiable and non-modifiable).

Non-modifiable factors	-Caucasian race -Thin constitution -Early menopause, amenorrhea -White skin and hair
Modifiable factors	-Smoker -Inactivity -Excessive alcohol consumption -Exercise-induced amenorrhea -Malnutrition and anorexia -Caffeine - High-fiber diet -Medications: glucocorticoids, thyroid hormones, diuretics, antiepileptics (phenytoin), benzodiazepines, antidepressants, heparin, methotrexate, *etc.*

Classification

Primary osteoporosis

Its cause is unknown.

Idiopathic or juvenile primary

It is detected in patients aged 8-14 years with osteopenia, growth retardation, and osteoarticular pain. Multiple microfractures can be seen in the vertebral bodies. Spontaneous resolution occurs 2-4 years after puberty.

Involutionary of the adult: There are 2 subtypes.

Postmenopausal (Type I)

It affects women with a frequency 6 times greater than men, aged 55-75 years. It is characterized by a rapid phase of osteoclast-mediated bone loss. It mainly affects cancellous bone and is associated with vertebral and distal radius fractures. Analytically, a decrease in PTH function and an increase in urinary calcium can be observed (frank hypercalciuria is detected in 20% of patients).

Senile (Type II)

It is related to aging (in women > 70 years and in men > 80 years). It affects women twice as often as men. It is produced by a decrease in osteoblastic activity and affects trabecular and cortical bone. It is characterized by vertebral and hip fractures.

Secondary osteoporosis

Its cause is known. There are several types:

• Drugs: heparin, antiestrogens, corticosteroids, methotrexate.

• Endocrine and metabolic diseases: hypogonadism, hyperparathyroidism, Cushing's disease, hyperthyroidism.

• Hematological: myeloma.

• Genetics: osteogenesis imperfecta, homocystinuria, Ehler-Danlos syndrome, and Marfan disease.

• Others: prolonged immobilization, mast cells, scurvy, malnutrition, alcoholism.

Clinical Presentation

It is usually asymptomatic until low energy or fragility fractures occur, being vertebral fractures the most frequent, specially located in the lumbar area. They produce sharp back pain that sometimes radiates to the abdomen, which intensifies when sitting down when standing up, and with the Valsalva maneuver. From a radiological point of view, there is an anterior collapse of the vertebral body that produces a decrease in height, dorsal kyphosis, and limited mobility of the spine.

Other common locations for osteoporotic fractures are the hip, distal forearm, and proximal humerus.

Diagnosis

It is based on densitometry (DEXA) and risk factors; there are no uniform diagnostic criteria in the world. Densitometry is the gold standard test. According to the WHO, osteoporosis is defined as a disease characterized by having a bone mineral density > 2.5 standard deviations below the maximum bone mass of a young person [3].

According to the densitometric result, the WHO classifies osteoporosis as follows (Table 2):

Table 2. Osteoporosis risks factors (modifiable and non-modifiable).

-	T value
NORMAL	-1 SD
OSTEOPENIA	Between -1 & -2'5
OSTEOPOROSIS	< -2'5
SEVERE OSTEOPOROSIS	< -2'5 + fracture

With the FRAX tool (Fracture Risk Assessment), the probability of suffering a fracture in the next 10 years can be estimated; an FRAX greater than or equal to 3% is considered a high risk of fracture.

SPINE SURGERY IN PATIENTS WITH OSTEOPOROSIS

Introduction

The number of people with osteoporosis is expected to increase more and more due to the increasing longevity of the population, so today's spine surgeons must know the influence of osteoporosis on the treatment of vertebral disorders.

Elderly patients maintain a high level of activity for a longer time than before, and their expectations regarding the proposed treatments are demanding. All these issues together with the advances made in surgical techniques and implants have led to more and more spinal surgeries being performed on the elderly population. Recent studies show that the expected survival after canal stenosis surgery in the elderly population is comparable to that observed in patients who undergo joint replacement [4, 5].

Osteoporosis predisposes the elderly patient to progressive spinal deformities and potential neurological compromise. The patient with osteoporosis is difficult to treat surgically due to both advanced age and the risks associated with anesthesia, making age sometimes be considered a relative contraindication for spinal surgery. The spine surgeon may need to address the direct sequelae of osteoporosis in the form of painful vertebral fractures and consequent deformity or may have to consider osteoporosis in relation to vertebral reconstructive surgery.

In patients with osteoporosis, certain principles must be observed:

1- Establish enough fixation points to provide good biomechanical stability.

2- Accept a lower degree of correction and not base the correction of the deformity on the implants used, but rather on ensuring adequate release of bone structures and soft parts.

3- Avoid ending fixation in kyphotic segments.

4- Try to re-establish, as far as possible, the spinopelvic parameters adapted to the patient's age.

Biomechanics of the Osteoporotic Spine

The vertebral body and the intervertebral disc support approximately 80% of the load during axial compression, the remaining 20% is supported by the facet joints [6]. The vertebral body is composed of a solid, surface-dense cortex and porous trabecular bone. As we get older, morphological and histological changes occur in the spine that increase the individual risk of injury. From the fourth decade of life, men can lose up to 30% and women 50% of their bone mineral density [7].

Osteoporosis can so weaken the bone structure that activities of daily living can exceed the load-bearing capacity of the vertebra. This weakness is not only due to the loss of bone mineral density but also due to changes in tissue microarchitecture or in the processes of remodeling and repair of microfractures. The vertebrae are the most frequently fractured bones in older people with osteoporosis. The type of vertebral fracture is related to the loss of bone mineral density and the lesion pattern, as well as the position of the spine at the time of the lesion [8].

Surgical Procedures in the Osteoporotic Spine

Vertebroplasty and Kyphoplasty

These are percutaneous spinal augmentation procedures. They are minimally invasive techniques for the treatment of osteoporotic vertebral fractures. They consist of the percutaneous injection guided by image techniques, of cement (polymethyl methacrylate or PMMA) inside the fractured vertebral body (Fig. **1**). Bone cement provides immediate stabilization of the fractured vertebral body, improving axial load capacity and pain relief. Numerous studies confirm the significant improvement after vertebroplasty or kyphoplasty in clinical symptoms caused by vertebral fracture, both in the short and the long term [9, 10].

Posterior Vertebral Instrumentation

Posterior vertebral instrumentation is used most often in the osteoporotic spine as a means of mechanical stabilization and as a promoter of arthrodesis after decompression of the neural elements. In this circumstance, the anterior column is typically intact and there is usually no significant instability, so posterior instrumentation in isolation is usually adequate. In addition, interbody arthrodesis implants in osteoporotic patients can cause endplate fracture and subsidence of the implant inside the vertebral body.

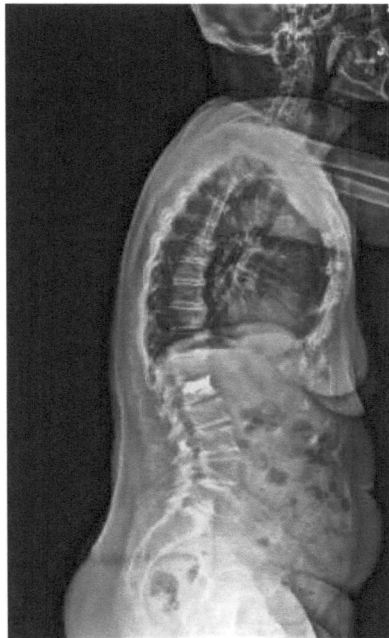

Fig. (1). L1 percutaneous vertebroplasty.

In current clinical practice, the vast majority of spinal surgeries with posterior instrumentation use pedicle screws, since they provide tricolumnar fixation. In the osteoporotic spine, the weak point in the assembly of the instrumentation is the contact surface between the implant and the bone; in this disease, the diameter of the intramedullary canal of the pedicle increases as the cortex gets thinner: this can make it difficult for the screws to achieve a proper bone purchase, causing gradual loosening of the implants, with resulting pseudoarthrosis and recurrence of the deformity [11, 12].

Posterior thoracolumbar instrumentation failure has been shown to correlate with BMD. Several studies have linked the linear correlation between the loss of pull-out resistance of pedicle screws as bone mineral density decreases [13, 14]. Failure in the osteoporotic spine is usually caused by the loss of screw fixation with cyclical loading, leading to loosening and eventually dislodgement of the implant. This can create a relatively large empty space around the loosened screw that prevents the same pedicle from being reused for a new re-instrumentation.

In order to try to improve the biomechanical conditions of the pedicle screws in this type of pathological bone, the surgeon has several options:

- Increasing the screw length: this increases resistance to screw pull-out, although this effect may be smaller in osteoporotic bone. The grip in the cortex is greater than in cancellous bone, so bicortical screws can increase the pull-out force by 20-50% [15]. However, bicortical fixation is usually only used at the S1 level due to the potential risk of damage to vascular structures located anterior to the vertebral bodies.
- Increasing the diameter of the screw: this also increases the resistance to cut off; however, the dimensions of the pedicle may limit the diameter of the screw. In the osteoporotic spine, when the screw diameter exceeds 70% of the pedicle diameter, the risk of pedicle fracture increases.
- Increasing the number of fixation levels: another strategy to improve the stability of the construct with pedicle screws in osteoporotic bone is to distribute the forces by increasing the number of fixation points to the spinal column. A balance must be made between the advantages offered by this option against the morbidity associated in the long term with the increase in the number of levels to be arthrodesed. It is important that the instrumentation does not end in a kyphotic segment, because progressive sagittal imbalance is a common problem in osteoporotic spine deformities and is the cause of instrument failure and fractures of adjacent levels.
- Adding sublaminar hooks to the pedicle screw assembly: sublaminar hooks are suitable for use in the osteoporotic spine because their fixation is in the relatively unaffected cortical lamellar bone. Biomechanical studies have confirmed the advantages offered by hybrid pedicle screws and sublaminar hook assemblies in increasing stiffness, pull-out resistance, and torsional stability in osteoporotic bone [16 - 18].
- Augmentation of pedicle screws: the contact surface between the bone and the screw can be improved by injecting PMMA bone cement through a fenestrated screw, it is what we call cemented pedicle screws. The administration of PMMA through this type of implant can increase the resistance to screw pull-out by 2 to 3 times.

- Use of cortical trajectory screws: Another instrumentation alternative in the degenerative pathology of the osteoporotic spine is the use of cortical trajectory screws. There are several works that propose these types of implants and routes as an alternative for fixation in patients with osteoporosis [19, 20].

CEMENTED PEDICLE SCREWS

Introduction

The surgical management of degenerative pathologies of the spine and vertebral fractures in patients with osteoporosis is a real challenge due to the peculiarities of this disease, as the loss of the trabecular microarchitecture of the vertebrae causes a decrease in the grip of the pedicle screws. To try to solve this problem, in recent decades, various surgical techniques have been developed that aim to increase the grip strength of pedicle screws. Among them, the most important is the development of cemented pedicle screws [21]. This is a type of distally fenestrated screw specifically designed for cement injection. Once the PMMA bone cement passes through the screw holes, by polymerization of the compound a continuous mass is formed between the screw shaft and the cancellous bone of the vertebral body. As a result, the cement provides immediate strength and rigidity and improves the grip of the screws.

Types of Implants

At the beginning of vertebral instrumentation with cement augmentation, bone cement was administered through vertebroplasty or kyphoplasty, to later proceed with the insertion of the screw [22, 23]. As pedicle screw designs evolved, perforated screws similar to those used in percutaneous surgery appeared. The mechanism by which the flow of cement accesses along the vertebra is through lateral holes in the screw shaft. Depending on the number of holes in the stem and their location, we can currently find different types of cemented pedicle screw designs [24 - 27] (Fig. **2**):

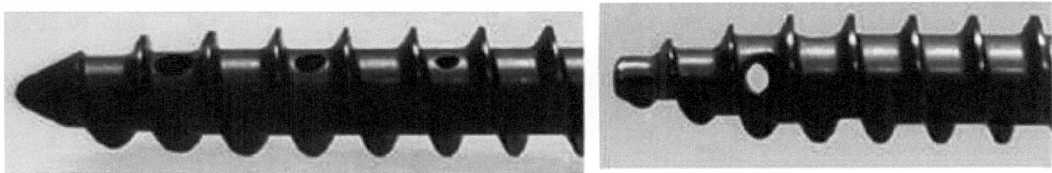

Fig. (2). Scattered and distal holes for augmented pedicle screws.

- screws with holes scattered throughout the stem: this increases the risk of intracanal leakage through inadvertent pedicle gaps.

- screws with holes close to the tip: allows a greater distribution of the cement in the anterior third of the body, which allows a better grip of the screw, and a lower rate of intracanal cement leakage.

Application of Cemented Pedicular Screws

There are numerous studies that demonstrate the advantages of using cemented pedicle screws for the treatment of degenerative pathology in the elderly with osteoporosis [28, 29], reducing the rate of screw loosening and the need for revision surgery compared to conventional ones [30].

Several studies have shown a higher fusion rate and lower risk of loosening of implants with cemented pedicle screws in osteoporotic bone compared to non-augmented implants [31, 32]. Additionally, there are no differences in the fusion or revision surgery rates between cemented posterolateral arthrodesis in patients over 75 years old and non-cemented posterolateral arthrodesis in patients under 65 years old [33].

Vertebral cementation with PMMA (polymethyl methacrylate) increases the pull-out force by approximately 150% compared to the initial force [34], improving deformity recurrence and increasing fusion rates for both. Some biomechanical studies carried out with this type of fenestrated screws have confirmed this resistance to pullout as well as a lower risk of implant breakage [35, 36]. The use of cemented fenestrated screws allows a more precise location of the cement and greater control over the release of the cement in the anterior third of the screw, thus reducing the risk of complications associated with cement leakage [37]. In a 2019 systematic review where the studies published to date regarding the use of cemented pedicle screws were analyzed [38], it was clear that their use is increasing for surgical treatment of the spine in patients with osteoporosis. Surgical indications in elderly patients are becoming more frequent, and the use of this augmentation technique improves the grip of the screws in this population and helps to maintain the clinical and radiological improvement obtained with surgery over time. This decreased risk of complications associated with the use of cemented screws in osteoporotic bone has also been confirmed by another recent meta-analysis.

It is important to use an adequate screw placement technique when using this type of implant, in order to achieve adequate distribution of the cement throughout the vertebral body. On the other hand, the best biomechanical conditions with the use of cemented pedicle screws are obtained when a symmetrical distribution of the cement mantle is achieved along the vertebral body [39]. However, this is not always possible and depends on other intrinsic factors of the patient such as their bone trabecular microarchitecture or the presence of vertebral sclerosis in the context of degenerative pathology. Some studies have also described the influence of the morphology of the vertebra according to its location in the spine on the spatial distribution of the cement around the screw [40]. In the case of the sacral vertebrae, the cement distribution is less homogeneous than with the lumbar ones.

The right moment to apply the cement is another controversial issue, especially if it is necessary to carry out a reduction maneuver through the fixation system. In elderly deformity surgeries, where it is required to apply reduction forces through the instrument, there are several screw-to-rod connection designs: top loading screws ("top loading"- rod connected to pedicle screw on top of long screw axis) or side loading ("side loading" - rod connected to pedicle screw on the side of the long screw axis). While the "top loading" systems force cementing before finishing assembling, the "side loading" systems allow cementing before or after this. Applying the cement before carrying out the reduction maneuvers would theoretically allow an increase in the force applied during the procedure, but there is an added risk of loosening the screw and cement below normal loading cycles. In contrast, cementation after having completed the reduction of the deformity prevents the application of greater force during maneuvers and can also cause trabecular fractures and loosening of the implant. However, subsequent cementation could reverse this initial biomechanical disadvantage. To analyze this issue further, a biomechanical study was carried out with 10 cadaveric lumbar vertebrae [41], observing that the pedicle screws that were cemented after reduction maneuvers fatigued after a greater number of loading cycles than those that were cemented prior to reduction. In addition, in case of post-reduction cementation, the loosening occurred in the assembly formed by the screw and the surrounding cement mantle. However, in the pre-reduction cementation group, the screw loosened within the cement mantle. After the implant failed, the mean displacement of the screw was the same in both groups. These findings allowed us to conclude that if a reduction maneuver is needed during osteoporotic bone deformity surgery, increasing the screws after reduction allows an improvement in the number of loading cycles necessary to loosen the implant and thus prevents an early assembly failure.

Biomaterials used in Vertebral Augmentation

Numerous screw augmentation materials have been proposed; among all of them, augmentation with PMMA cement (Fig. **3**) seems to be the most effective method according to the findings of biomechanical studies. The use of a second generation of perforated pedicle screws with the new forms of PMMA has probably been the cause of this improvement compared to the first studies carried out with this type of cement. In a biomechanical study carried out on cadavers [42], the superiority of PMMA in pull-out resistance was observed with respect to controls, hydroxyapatite, and calcium phosphate. The latter also improves the contact surface between the screw and the bone and therefore improves resistance to pullout. This cement has a compressive strength between that of cancellous and cortical bone but has a shear and tensile strength lower than that of cancellous bone. Moore *et al.* [43] compared, in a cadaver study, the biomechanical properties of PMMA cement and calcium phosphate cement: the increase in pull-out force with PMMA cementation was 147%, compared to 102% with calcium phosphate cement. They also described different screw failure mechanisms between augmentation with PMMA and calcium phosphate in the stress tests performed: with PMMA, implant failure was caused by a fracture of the pedicle at or near its junction with the vertebral body in 80% (25 of 30) of the samples, whilst on the contrary, implant failure with calcium phosphate occurred most frequently at the interface between the cement and the screw in 80% (24 of 30) of the samples.

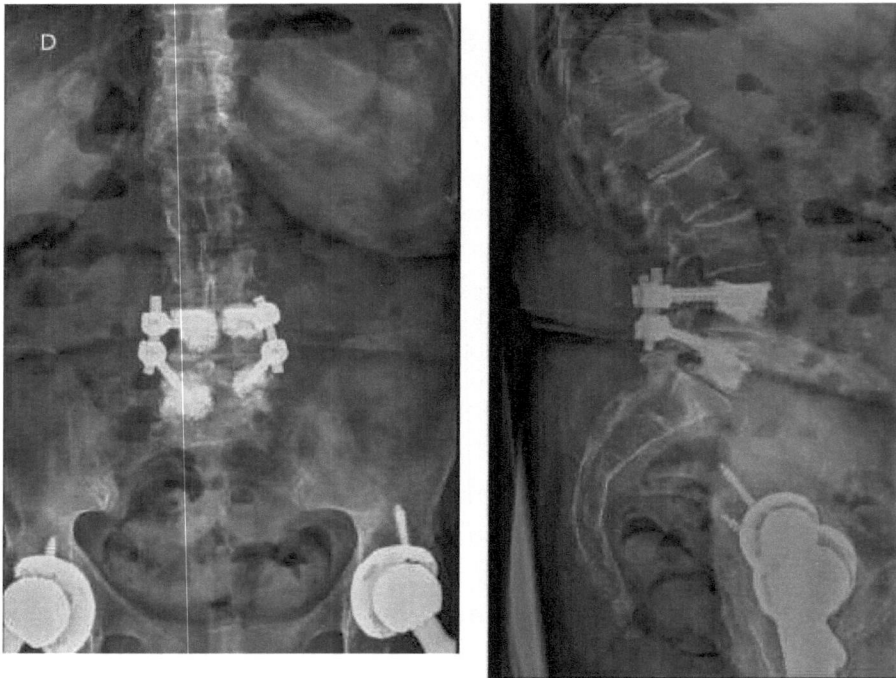

Fig. (3). Example of L4-5 cemented screws.

Although PMMA cement has been used for many years and has proven its efficacy, it has some drawbacks that foster the creation of new lines of research with other biomaterials for use in screw augmentation. Among the disadvantages described for PMMA [44], we find the exothermic reaction that generates its polymerization, the lack of biodegradability and osteoconductivity, the toxicity of the monomer used, and the limited working time.

Another option is the usage of hydroxyapatite coating of the screws, which has biological advantages of promoting bone growth and being biodegradable, with superior grip strength compared to uncoated screws [45]. However, the difficulty of extraction with this type of implant when this is required in revision surgery has been described as an important disadvantage. In a prospective, randomized, unblinded clinical trial, hydroxyapatite-coated pedicle screws were compared with uncoated screws, and it was found that the torque required to remove them in revision surgeries was significantly higher in the hydroxyapatite group [46]. This fact is especially relevant in the case of osteoporotic bones where complications such as bone defects and fractures can occur during the extraction process.

Other types of biological cements are being investigated, such as polydicalcium phosphate dihydrate (P-DCPD) [47]. This compound, still under investigation, would have the theoretical advantage over the already known PMMA, which would not undergo an exothermic reaction and would improve the dissolution capacity of drugs, useful in certain situations.

COMPLICATIONS WITH THE USE OF CEMENTED PEDICULAR SCREWS

Like any other surgical technique or when any implant is used, there are several risks and complications that we must take into account when indicating them. Regarding the use of pedicle screws, the most frequent complications to consider are: cement leakage, infection, and possible difficulty in extracting the screws if necessary in the future.

In a study [48], where a total of 1043 instrumented vertebrae with cemented pedicle screws were analyzed, a cement leakage rate of up to 62.3% was described, without any major associated complications. 0.6% of the patients who suffered a leak presented radicular pain secondary to the presence of cement in the foramen. On the other hand, among the patients who required revision surgery, there were no problems during the removal of the screws.

Cement Leak

Extravertebral cement leakage is the most frequent complication; this is usually asymptomatic, however, there are cases of serious complications and death reported in the literature. Complications due to cement leaks outside the vertebral body include pulmonary embolism ([49, 50]), cement in the vena cava, heart, and kidneys, spinal cord compression when the leak is into the vertebral canal, and foraminal leak with root compression. The rate of cement leakage during augmentation techniques varies between 5-80% [51, 52]; however, this figure increases to 63-87% when analyzed with postoperative CT instead of plain radiography [53 - 55]. The biggest theoretical problem found with cement leakage is the potential risk of neural damage caused by either the exothermic reaction of PMMA or by mechanical compression. However, the presence of cement in the foramen or epidural space, in clinical practice, rarely produces any neurological damage.

There are different patterns of cement leakage described according to the classification proposed by Yeom *et al.* [56] (Fig. **4**):

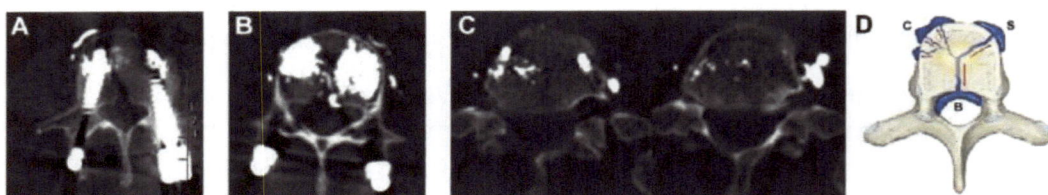

Fig. (4). Different patterns of cement leakage. **A**: segmental; **B**: basivertebral; **C**: cortical; **D**: comparison among them.

- Type S: Cement leak through the **S**egmental vein pathway.
- Type B: Leakage of cement through the **B**asivertebral vein, which in the spinal canal is dispersed through the venous epidural plexus.
- Type C: Leakage of cement through a break or defect in the **C**ortical wall.

One of the most frequent areas of leakage is the lateral venous system. Osteoporotic vertebral fractures not only increase the leak occurrence in comparison with degenerative pathology, but also the existence of vertebral collapse changes the pattern of cement leakage, increasing the incidence of type B leaks [57, 58].

Another important issue with cement leaks is the risk of fractures at adjacent vertebrae. The presence of leaks in the intradiscal space has been related to a significant increase in the incidence of new fractures in adjacent vertebral bodies [59].

There is some controversy as to whether the volume of cement administered could influence the risk of leakage. There are authors who argue that the lower the volume of cement, the less risk of leakage [60]. It is also true that a smaller amount of cement could also decrease the resistance to pull-out. However, some studies [61] found no statistically significant differences regarding screw resistance between administering a total of 1 mL of cement per vertebra *versus* 3 mL. Other authors relate the risk of leakage not to the volume of cement administered, but rather to the patient's bone quality, with a positive association between the risk of leakage and low bone mineral density. To reduce the risk of leakage, the use of high-viscosity cement [62, 63] or the sequential and slow injection of small volumes of cement [64] is recommended.

Infection

One of the concerns regarding the use of PMMA in instrumented spinal surgery is the potential risk of infection, where the presence of cement can make infection management difficult. In this regard, the risk of infection is low according to studies that analyzed vertebroplasties performed in elderly people with risk factors for infection [65]. When it occurs, aggressive washing and debridement of the surgical wound associated with antibiotic therapy is usually sufficient, without the need to remove the implants in most cases.

Implant Removal

The removal of cemented pedicle screws can be a problem in revision surgery, especially in the case of brittle osteoporotic bone. Biomechanical studies have analyzed this complication. Cho *et al.* found that PMMA-augmented pedicle screws can be easily and safely removed. However, the torque required to remove them is greater than in the case of non-cemented screws [66, 67]. No relationship has been observed between the torsion force required for its extraction and the volume of cement administered.

The clinical studies carried out also confirm the absence of clinically relevant difficulty in removing cemented pedicle screws in revision surgeries with osteoporotic bone, advising in use whenever it's necessary.

CONCLUSION

The number of people with osteoporosis is expected to increase. Osteoporosis predisposes elderly patients to progressive spinal deformities and potential neurological compromise. Several surgical procedures can be performed to treat the osteoporotic spine, including vertebroplasty, kyphoplasty, and posterior vertebral instrumentation. In order to improve the biomechanical conditions of the pedicle screws in this type of pathological bone, we can increase the screw length, diameter, and the number of fixation levels, or use cemented pedicle screws. This involves a distally fenestrated screw specifically designed for cement injection (PMMA). Numerous studies demonstrate the advantages of using cemented pedicle screws for the treatment of degenerative pathology in the elderly with osteoporosis. This approach reduces the rate of screw loosening and the need for revision surgery compared to conventional ones. However, there are some complications related to the use of cemented pedicular screws such as cement leakage, infection, or challenges in revision surgeries.

REFERENCES

[1]   Tomé-Bermejo F, Piñera AR, Álvarez-Galovich L. Osteoporosis and the management of spinal degenerative disease (I). Arch Bone Jt Surg 2017; 5(5): 272-82.
        [PMID: 29226197]

[2]   Hernlund E, Svedbom A, Ivergård M, *et al.* Osteoporosis in the European Union: medical management, epidemiology and economic burden. Arch Osteoporos 2013; 8(1-2): 136.
        [http://dx.doi.org/10.1007/s11657-013-0136-1] [PMID: 24113837]

[3]   Ritter MA, Albohm MJ, Keating EM, Faris PM, Meding JB. Life expectancy after total hip arthroplasty. J Arthroplasty 1998; 13(8): 874-5.
        [http://dx.doi.org/10.1016/S0883-5403(98)90192-9] [PMID: 9880178]

[4]   Schrøder HM, Kristensen PW, Petersen MB, Nielsen PT. Patient survival after total knee arthroplasty: 5-year data in 926 patients. Acta Orthop Scand 1998; 69(1): 35-8.
        [http://dx.doi.org/10.3109/17453679809002353] [PMID: 9524515]

[5]   Ponnusamy KE, Iyer S, Gupta G, Khanna AJ. Instrumentation of the osteoporotic spine: biomechanical and clinical considerations. Spine J 2011; 11(1): 54-63.
        [http://dx.doi.org/10.1016/j.spinee.2010.09.024] [PMID: 21168099]

[6]   White A, Panjabi M. Clinical biomechanics of the spine 2nd ed., 1990.

[7]   Mazess RB. On aging bone loss. Clin Orthop Relat Res 1982; (165): 239-52.
        [PMID: 7075066]

[8]   Bono CM, Einhorn TA. Overview of osteoporosis: pathophysiology and determinants of bone strength. Eur Spine J 2003; 12(0) (Suppl. 2): S90-6.
        [http://dx.doi.org/10.1007/s00586-003-0603-2] [PMID: 13680312]

[9]   Sanli I, van Kuijk SMJ, de Bie RA, van Rhijn LW, Willems PC. Percutaneous cement augmentation in the treatment of osteoporotic vertebral fractures (OVFs) in the elderly: a systematic review. Eur Spine J 2020; 29(7): 1553-72.
        [http://dx.doi.org/10.1007/s00586-020-06391-x] [PMID: 32240375]

[10]   Anderson PA, Froyshteter AB, Tontz WL Jr. Meta-analysis of vertebral augmentation compared with conservative treatment for osteoporotic spinal fractures. J Bone Miner Res 2013; 28(2): 372-82.
        [http://dx.doi.org/10.1002/jbmr.1762] [PMID: 22991246]

[11]   Jost B, Cripton PA, Lund T, *et al.* Compressive strength of interbody cages in the lumbar spine: the effect of cage shape, posterior instrumentation and bone density. Eur Spine J 1998; 7(2): 132-41.
        [http://dx.doi.org/10.1007/s005860050043] [PMID: 9629937]

[12]   Andersen T, Christensen FB, Niedermann B, Helmig P, Høy K, Hansen ES, *et al.* Impact of instrumentation in followed for 2-7 years. Acta Orthop 2009; 80(4): 445-50.
        [http://dx.doi.org/10.3109/17453670903170505] [PMID: 19626471]

[13]   Yagi M, Ogiri M, Holy CE, Bourcet A. Comparison of clinical effectiveness of fenestrated and conventional pedicle screws in patients undergoing spinal surgery: a systematic review and meta-analysis. Expert Rev Med Devices 2021; 18(10): 995-1022.
        [http://dx.doi.org/10.1080/17434440.2021.1977123] [PMID: 34503387]

[14]   Polly DW Jr, Orchowski JR, Ellenbogen RG. Revision pedicle screws. Bigger, longer shims--what is best? Spine 1998; 23(12): 1374-9.
        [http://dx.doi.org/10.1097/00007632-199806150-00015] [PMID: 9654629]

[15]   Zindrick MR, Wiltse LL, Widell EH, *et al.* A biomechanical study of intrapeduncular screw fixation in the lumbosacral spine. Clin Orthop Relat Res 1986; 203(&NA;): 99-112.
[http://dx.doi.org/10.1097/00003086-198602000-00012] [PMID: 3956001]

[16]   Hasegawa K, Takahashi HE, Uchiyama S, *et al.* An experimental study of a combination method using a pedicle screw and laminar hook for the osteoporotic spine. Spine 1997; 22(9): 958-62.
[http://dx.doi.org/10.1097/00007632-199705010-00004] [PMID: 9152444]

[17]   Coe JD, Warden KE, Herzig MA, McAfee PC. Influence of bone mineral density on the fixation of thoracolumbar implants. A comparative study of transpedicular screws, laminar hooks, and spinous process wires. Spine (PhilaPa 1976) 1990; 15(9): 902-7.
[http://dx.doi.org/10.1097/00007632-199009000-00012] [PMID: 2259978]

[18]   Liljenqvist U, Hackenberg L, Link T, Halm H. Pullout strength of pedicle screws *versus* pedicle and laminar hooks in the thoracic spine. Acta Orthop Belg 2001; 67(2): 157-63.
[PMID: 11383294]

[19]   Ding H, Hai Y, Liu Y, *et al.* Cortical trajectory fixation *versus* traditional pedicle-screw fixation in the treatment of lumbar degenerative patients with osteoporosis: a prospective randomized controlled trial. Clin Interv Aging 2022; 17: 175-84.
[http://dx.doi.org/10.2147/CIA.S349533] [PMID: 35237030]

[20]   Song T, Hsu WK, Ye T. Lumbar pedicle cortical bone trajectory screw. Chin Med J (Engl) 2014; 127(21): 3808-13.
[http://dx.doi.org/10.3760/cma.j.issn.0366-6999.20141887] [PMID: 25382340]

[21]   Zhang J, Wang G, Zhang N. A meta-analysis of complications associated with the use of cement-augmented pedicle screws in osteoporosis of spine. Orthop Traumatol Surg Res 2021; 107(7): 102791.
[http://dx.doi.org/10.1016/j.otsr.2020.102791] [PMID: 33338677]

[22]   Linhardt O, Lüring C, Matussek J, Hamberger C, Plitz W, Grifka J. Stability of pedicle screws after kyphoplasty augmentation: an experimental study to compare transpedicular screw fixation in soft and cured kyphoplasty cement. J Spinal Disord Tech 2006; 19(2): 87-91.
[http://dx.doi.org/10.1097/01.bsd.0000177212.52583.bd] [PMID: 16760780]

[23]   Becker S, Chavanne A, Spitaler R, *et al.* Assessment of different screw augmentation techniques and screw designs in osteoporotic spines. Eur Spine J 2008; 17(11): 1462-9.
[http://dx.doi.org/10.1007/s00586-008-0769-8] [PMID: 18781342]

[24]   Yang K, You Y, Wu W. The influence of different injection hole designs of augmented pedicle screws on bone cement leakage and distribution patterns in osteoporotic patients. World Neurosurg 2022; 157: e40-8.
[http://dx.doi.org/10.1016/j.wneu.2021.09.086] [PMID: 34583006]

[25]   Amendola L, Gasbarrini A, Fosco M, *et al.* Fenestrated pedicle screws for cement-augmented purchase in patients with bone softening: a review of 21 cases. J Orthop Traumatol 2011; 12(4): 193-9.
[http://dx.doi.org/10.1007/s10195-011-0164-9] [PMID: 22065147]

[26]   Chang MC, Liu CL, Chen TH. Polymethylmethacrylate augmentation of pedicle screw for osteoporotic spinal surgery: a novel technique. Spine (PhilaPa 1976) 2008; 3310: E317-24.
[http://dx.doi.org/10.1097/BRS.0b013e31816f6c73] [PMID: 18449032]

[27]   Hu MH, Wu HTH, Chang MC, Yu WK, Wang ST, Liu CL. Polymethylmethacrylate augmentation of the pedicle screw: the cement distribution in the vertebral body. Eur Spine J 2011; 20(8): 1281-8.
[http://dx.doi.org/10.1007/s00586-011-1824-4] [PMID: 21533852]

[28]   Alvarez-Galovich L, Tome-Bermejo F, Moya AB, *et al.* Safety and efficacy with augmented second-generation perforated pedicle screws in treating degenerative spine disease in elderly population. Int J Spine Surg 2020; 14(5): 811-7.
[http://dx.doi.org/10.14444/7115] [PMID: 33097578]

[29]   Piñera AR, Duran C, Lopez B, Saez I, Correia E, Alvarez L. Instrumented lumbar arthrodesis in

elderly patients: prospective study using cannulated cemented pedicle screw instrumentation. Eur Spine J 2011; 3: 408-14.
[http://dx.doi.org/10.1007/s00586-011-1907-2] [PMID: 21850421] [PMCID: 3175826]

[30]   Yagi M, Ogiri M, Holy CE, Bourcet A. Comparison of clinical effectiveness of fenestrated and conventional pedicle screws in patients undergoing spinal surgery: a systematic review and meta-analysis. Expert Rev Med Devices 2021; 18(10): 995-1022.
[http://dx.doi.org/10.1080/17434440.2021.1977123] [PMID: 34503387]

[31]   Wang Y, Zhou C, Yin H, Song D. Comparison of cement-augmented pedicle screw and conventional pedicle screw for the treatment of lumbar degenerative patients with osteoporosis. Eur J Orthop Surg Traumatol 2024; 34(3): 1609-17.
[http://dx.doi.org/10.1007/s00590-024-03849-2] [PMID: 38363348]

[32]   Sawakami K, Yamazaki A, Ishikawa S, Ito T, Watanabe K, Endo N. Polymethylmethacrylate augmentation of pedicle screws increases the initial fixation in osteoporotic spine patients. J Spinal Disord Tech 2012; 25(2): E28-35.
[http://dx.doi.org/10.1097/BSD.0b013e318228bbed] [PMID: 22454185]

[33]   Tomé-Bermejo F, Moreno-Mateo F, Piñera-Parrilla Á, *et al.* Instrumented lumbar fusion in patients over 75 years of age: is it worthwhile?—a comparative study of the improvement in quality of life between elderly and young patients. J Spine Surg 2023; 9(3): 247-58.
[http://dx.doi.org/10.21037/jss-22-115] [PMID: 37841795]

[34]   Pfeifer BA, Krag MH, Johnson C. Repair of failed transpedicle screw fixation. A biomechanical study comparing polymethylmethacrylate, milled bone, and matchstick bone reconstruction. Spine 1994; 19(3): 350-3.
[http://dx.doi.org/10.1097/00007632-199402000-00017] [PMID: 8171370]

[35]   Elder BD, Lo SFL, Holmes C, *et al.* The biomechanics of pedicle screw augmentation with cement. Spine J 2015; 15(6): 1432-45.
[http://dx.doi.org/10.1016/j.spinee.2015.03.016] [PMID: 25797809]

[36]   Schulze M, Riesenbeck O, Vordemvenne T, *et al.* Complex biomechanical properties of non-augmented and augmented pedicle screws in human vertebrae with reduced bone density. BMC Musculoskelet Disord 2020; 21(1): 151.
[http://dx.doi.org/10.1186/s12891-020-3158-z] [PMID: 32143605]

[37]   Lehman, Ronald A. Jr MD; Kang, Daniel Gene MD; Wagner, Scott Cameron MD. Management of osteoporosis in spine surgery. Journal of the American Academy of Orthopaedic Surgeons 2015; 23(4): 253-63.
[http://dx.doi.org/10.5435/JAAOS-D-14-00042]

[38]   Singh V, Mahajan R, Das K, Chhabra HS, Rustagi T. Surgical trend analysis for use of cement augmented pedicle screws in osteoporosis of spine: a systematic review (2000-2017). Global Spine J 2019; 9(7): 783-95.
[http://dx.doi.org/10.1177/2192568218801570] [PMID: 31552160]

[39]   Wittenberg RH, Lee KS, Shea M, White AA III, Hayes WC. Effect of screw diameter, insertion technique, and bone cement augmentation of pedicular screw fixation strength. Clin Orthop Relat Res 1993; 296(296): 278-87.
[http://dx.doi.org/10.1097/00003086-199311000-00045] [PMID: 8222439]

[40]   González SG, Bastida GC, Vlad MD, *et al.* Analysis of bone cement distribution around fenestrated pedicle screws in low bone quality lumbosacral vertebrae. Int Orthop 2019; 43(8): 1873-82.
[http://dx.doi.org/10.1007/s00264-018-4115-4] [PMID: 30141139]

[41]   Schmoelz W, Heinrichs CH, Schmidt S, *et al.* Timing of PMMA cement application for pedicle screw augmentation affects screw anchorage. Eur Spine J 2017; 26(11): 2883-90.
[http://dx.doi.org/10.1007/s00586-017-5053-3] [PMID: 28374330]

[42]   Yi S, Rim DC, Park SW, Murovic JA, Lim J, Park J. Biomechanical comparisons of pull out strengths

after pedicle screw augmentation with hydroxyapatite, calcium phosphate, or polymethylmethacrylate in the cadaveric spine. World Neurosurg 2015; 83(6): 976-81.
[http://dx.doi.org/10.1016/j.wneu.2015.01.056] [PMID: 25769482]

[43] Moore DC, Maitra RS, Farjo LA, Graziano GP, Goldstein SA. Restoration of pedicle screw fixation with an *in situ* setting calcium phosphate cement. Spine (PhilaPa 1976) 1997; 22(15): 1696-705.
[http://dx.doi.org/10.1097/00007632-199708010-00003] [PMID: 9259778]

[44] Sun H, Liu C, Chen S, *et al.* Effect of surgical factors on the augmentation of cement-injectable cannulated pedicle screw fixation by a novel calcium phosphate-based nanocomposite. Front Med 2019; 13(5): 590-601.
[http://dx.doi.org/10.1007/s11684-019-0710-z] [PMID: 31555965]

[45] Deligianni D, Korovessis P, Porte-Derrieu MC, Amedee J. Fibronectin preadsorbed on hydroxyapatite together with rough surface structure increases osteoblasts' adhesion "*in vitro*": the theoretical usefulness of fibronectin preadsorption on hydroxyapatite to increase permanent stability and longevity in spine implants. J Spinal Disord Tech 2005; 18(3): 257-62.
[PMID: 15905771]

[46] Sandén B, Olerud C, Petrén-Mallmin M, Larsson S. Hydroxyapatite coating improves fixation of pedicle screws. J Bone Joint Surg Br 2002; 84-B(3): 387-91.
[http://dx.doi.org/10.1302/0301-620X.84B3.0840387] [PMID: 12002498]

[47] Criado A, Yokhana S, Rahman T, *et al.* Biomechanical strength comparison of pedicle screw augmentation using poly-dicalcium phosphate dihydrate (P-DCPD) and polymethylmethacrylate (PMMA) cements. Spine Deform 2020; 8(2): 165-70.
[http://dx.doi.org/10.1007/s43390-019-00022-2] [PMID: 32030639]

[48] Martín-Fernández M, López-Herradón A, Piñera AR, *et al.* Potential risks of using cement-augmented screws for spinal fusion in patients with low bone quality. Spine J 2017; 17(8): 1192-9.
[http://dx.doi.org/10.1016/j.spinee.2017.04.029] [PMID: 28606606]

[49] Guo H, Tang Y, Guo D, *et al.* The cement leakage in cement-augmented pedicle screw instrumentation in degenerative lumbosacral diseases: a retrospective analysis of 202 cases and 950 augmented pedicle screws. Eur Spine J 2019; 28(7): 1661-9.
[http://dx.doi.org/10.1007/s00586-019-05985-4] [PMID: 31030261]

[50] Janssen I, Ryang YM, Gempt J, *et al.* Risk of cement leakage and pulmonary embolism by bone cement-augmented pedicle screw fixation of the thoracolumbar spine. Spine J 2017; 17(6): 837-44.
[http://dx.doi.org/10.1016/j.spinee.2017.01.009] [PMID: 28108403]

[51] Hulme PA, Krebs J, Ferguson SJ, Berlemann U. Vertebroplasty and kyphoplasty: a systematic review of 69 clinical studies. Spine 2006; 31(17): 1983-2001.
[http://dx.doi.org/10.1097/01.brs.0000229254.89952.6b] [PMID: 16924218]

[52] Schmidt R, Cakir B, Mattes T, Wegener M, Puhl W, Richter M. Cement leakage during vertebroplasty: an underestimated problem? Eur Spine J 2005; 14(5): 466-73.
[http://dx.doi.org/10.1007/s00586-004-0839-5] [PMID: 15690210]

[53] Muijs SPJ, Akkermans PA, van Erkel AR, Dijkstra SD. The value of routinely performing a bone biopsy during percutaneous vertebroplasty in treatment of osteoporotic vertebral compression fractures. Spine 2009; 34(22): 2395-9.
[http://dx.doi.org/10.1097/BRS.0b013e3181b8707e] [PMID: 19829253]

[54] Álvarez L, Alcaraz M, Pérez-Higueras A, *et al.* Percutaneous vertebroplasty: functional improvement in patients with osteoporotic compression fractures. Spine 2006; 31(10): 1113-8.
[http://dx.doi.org/10.1097/01.brs.0000216487.97965.38] [PMID: 16648745]

[55] Yeom JS, Kim WJ, Choy WS, Lee CK, Chang BS, Kang JW. Leakage of cement in percutaneous transpedicular vertebroplasty for painful osteoporotic compression fractures. J Bone Joint Surg Br 2003; 85-B(1): 83-9.
[http://dx.doi.org/10.1302/0301-620X.85B1.13026] [PMID: 12585583]

[56]   Álvarez L, Pérez-Higueras A, Granizo JJ, de Miguel I, Quiñones D, Rossi RE. Predictors of outcomes of percutaneous vertebroplasty for osteoporotic vertebral fractures. Spine 2005; 30(1): 87-92.
[http://dx.doi.org/10.1097/00007632-200501010-00016] [PMID: 15626987]

[57]   Lee IJ, Choi AL, Yie MY, *et al.* CT evaluation of local leakage of bone cement after percutaneous kyphoplasty and vertebroplasty. Acta Radiol 2010; 51(6): 649-54.
[http://dx.doi.org/10.3109/02841851003620366] [PMID: 20528649]

[58]   Tomé-Bermejo F, Piñera AR, Duran-Álvarez C, *et al.* Identification of risk factors for the occurrence of cement leakage during percutaneous vertebroplasty for painful osteoporotic or malignant vertebral fracture. Spine 2014; 39(11): E693-700.
[http://dx.doi.org/10.1097/BRS.0000000000000294] [PMID: 24583722]

[59]   Lin EP, Ekholm S, Hiwatashi A, Westesson PL. Vertebroplasty: cement leakage into the disc increases the risk of new fracture of adjacent vertebral body. AJNR Am J Neuroradiol 2004; 25(2): 175-80.
[PMID: 14970015]

[60]   Guo H, Tang Y, Guo D, *et al.* The cement leakage in cement-augmented pedicle screw instrumentation in degenerative lumbosacral diseases: a retrospective analysis of 202 cases and 950 augmented pedicle screws. Eur Spine J 2019; 28(7): 1661-9.
[http://dx.doi.org/10.1007/s00586-019-05985-4] [PMID: 31030261]

[61]   Weiser L, Sellenschloh K, Püschel K, *et al.* Reduced cement volume does not affect screw stability in augmented pedicle screws. Eur Spine J 2020; 29(6): 1297-303.
[http://dx.doi.org/10.1007/s00586-020-06376-w] [PMID: 32206868]

[62]   Zhang L, Wang J, Feng X, *et al.* A comparison of high viscosity bone cement and low viscosity bone cement vertebroplasty for severe osteoporotic vertebral compression fractures. Clin Neurol Neurosurg 2015; 129: 10-6.
[http://dx.doi.org/10.1016/j.clineuro.2014.11.018] [PMID: 25524481]

[63]   La Maida GA, Giarratana LS, Acerbi A, Ferrari V, Mineo GV, Misaggi B. Cement leakage: safety of minimally invasive surgical techniques in the treatment of multiple myeloma vertebral lesions. Eur Spine J 2012; 21(S1) (Suppl. 1): 61-8.
[http://dx.doi.org/10.1007/s00586-012-2221-3] [PMID: 22411037]

[64]   Hoppe S, Wangler S, Aghayev E, Gantenbein B, Boger A, Benneker LM. Reduction of cement leakage by sequential PMMA application in a vertebroplasty model. Eur Spine J 2016; 25(11): 3450-5.
[http://dx.doi.org/10.1007/s00586-015-3920-3] [PMID: 25841359]

[65]   Abdelrahman H, Siam AE, Shawky A, Ezzati A, Boehm H. Infection after vertebroplasty or kyphoplasty. A series of nine cases and review of literature. Spine J 2013; 13(12): 1809-17.
[http://dx.doi.org/10.1016/j.spinee.2013.05.053] [PMID: 23880354]

[66]   Cho W, Wu C, Zheng X, *et al.* Is it safe to back out pedicle screws after augmentation with polymethyl methacrylate or calcium phosphate cement? A biomechanical study. J Spinal Disord Tech 2011; 24(4): 276-9.
[http://dx.doi.org/10.1097/BSD.0b013e3181f605d0] [PMID: 20975600]

[67]   Bullmann V, Schmoelz W, Richter M, Grathwohl C, Schulte TL. Revision of cannulated and perforated cement-augmented pedicle screws: a biomechanical study in human cadavers. Spine 2010; 35(19): E932-9.
[http://dx.doi.org/10.1097/BRS.0b013e3181c6ec60] [PMID: 20508553]

CHAPTER 5

Degenerative Spondylolisthesis: Why Does it Occur and How the Body Reacts?

Enrique Marescot-Rodríguez[1], Máximo-Alberto Díez-Ulloa[2,*], Luis Puente-Sánchez[2], Eva Díez-Sanchidrián[3] and Javier Melchor Duart-Clemente[4]

[1] *Orthopedics Department, Pontevedra University Hospital, Pontevedra, Spain*

[2] *Spinal Unit, Orthopedics Department, University Hospital Complex of Santiago de Compostela, Santiago, Spain*

[3] *Faculty of Medicine, Santiago de Compostela University, Santiago, Spain*

[4] *Neurosurgery and Spinal Surgery Departments, Valencia General Hospital, Valencia, Spain*

Abstract: Degenerative spondylolisthesis (DS) is a common entity in the fifth-sixth decade of life, and it is assumed that there is a biomechanical rationale behind the pathogeny as it will not develop in all individuals. There are several causes that could initiate its natural history: strong lumbopelvic anatomical fixations, ligamentous laxity, sarcopenia, spinopelvic parameters, *etc*. In the end, it will stabilize by itself due to the Kirkaldy-Willis cycle. The issue arises when it becomes symptomatic because of the facet deformity and hypertrophy together with the endplate spondylotic osteophytes - even with small displacements-, producing a central and lateral stenosis with a concomitant pluriradicular involvement. The biomechanical background is analyzed to provide clues to understand the natural history of DS and set the rationale for treatment.

Keywords: Pelvic incidence, Spondylolisthesis, Spondylolysis, Spinal balance.

INTRODUCTION

Degenerative spondylolisthesis (DS) is diagnosed when there is a ventral displacement of one vertebra over the adjacent one without affecting the integrity of the posterior structures. It could be understood as a rupture or insufficiency of the spine in two when it fails due to a concentration of stresses at this level that results in the anterior sliding of (most frequently) L4 over L5, due to instability in the lumbar segment; this concentration of tensions is due to the fixation of L5 to the pelvis by strong iliotransverse ligaments, transmitting the anterior shearing tensions in the flexion-extension movements to the immediately superior disc (L4-L5).

* **Corresponding author Máximo-Alberto Díez-Ulloa:** Spinal Unit, Orthopedics Department, University Hospital Complex of Santiago de Compostela, Santiago, Spain; E-mail: maximoalberto.diez@usc.es

Javier Melchor Duart Clemente (Ed.)

This fact has promoted the study of possible causes that may explain the beginning of this particular displacement, among them:

1. Lack of ligamentous laxity, supported mainly by the fact that it is more frequent in women (1:3 ratio in the Framingham Heart Study) of middle age with estrogen deficiency; patients with estrogen receptor alpha deficiency have a higher prevalence of DS [1].
2. Degenerative disc disease (DDD). The loss of hydrostatic pressure of the disk causes a loss of height and a loss of resistance to displacement with shearing. The start of the degenerative cascade in the intervertebral disc and posterior articular facets causes instability of the mobile vertebral segment that can lead to the development of DDD (one study shows the disease of several disc segments in the context of DS) [2]. The vertebral segment in which this lesion most frequently occurs is L4-L5 and there are certain anatomical conditions at that level that can facilitate the onset and development of this pathology, among them the inclination of the upper vertebral plate of L4 at more than $10°$ with respect to the horizontal or the sagittal orientation of the articular facets, with interfacetal angles greater than $60°$ (although this association is not clear whether it may be a cause or a consequence) [3].
3. The morphology of the distal segments of the vertebral spine and their relationship to the pelvis, including the strong iliotransverse ligaments. Biomechanical factors would be especially relevant including all those that facilitate an anterior displacement of the center of gravity, such as obesity [4]. In this line, it would be worth studying the distribution of shapes of the spine (following Roussouly) [5] with the two arches of lumbar lordosis, divided precisely by the upper plate of L4, which is assumed to be parallel to the ground.

ETIOPATHOGENESIS

The cause of DS is currently unknown, and many etiological factors have been implicated, so the general opinion is that its cause is multifactorial.

Both local anatomical factors and others of a more general nature that favor the degenerative displacement of one vertebra over another could be taken into account. Among these local factors, it has been found that there is a molding towards the sagittalization in the arrangement of the articular facets of the L4-L5 joint secondary to destabilization due to disc degeneration and the concentration of shear stresses at that level. In this situation, they would offer less resistance to the anterior displacement of one vertebral body over another, to which ligamentous laxity would also help. On the other hand, there are more general factors mainly of a biomechanical nature that favor this displacement, including a greater inclination of the L4 vertebral body and the different values of spinopelvic parameters in patients suffering from DDD in relation to the healthy population.

In the L4-L5 segment, two important biomechanical situations are combined so that it is precisely at this point where the pathology develops: a) it is the most mobile segment of the lumbar spine, and therefore, more susceptible to becoming unstable; and b) the total lordosis of the lumbar spine is considered to be formed by two arches, an upper one (related to thoracic kyphosis) and a lower one -in which two-thirds of the global lordosis are located- and that the inflection point of those arches happens to meet at the L4 superior vertebral endplate, which presupposes that the facet joints at that level possibly bear relevant stress forces. Together with this, there is a more "stable" disposition of L5 due to its embedded position in the pelvis, fixed by powerful iliolumbar ligaments and by its posterior articulations with S1, generally oriented in the coronal plane. Thus, we speak of "deeply seated" L5 vertebrae, as a predisposing factor to DS.

The influence of the force vectors that -as noted above- affect this segment, can facilitate its instability and the progression towards DS. Therefore, it is pertinent to study the relationship of the lumbar region with the pelvis, through the spinopelvic parameters. A more inclined glide plane will favor the ventral displacement of the L4 vertebral body over that of L5. This "favorable" condition is typically found in those spines with a lordosis of greater magnitude both in its absolute value and in the number of segments involved in it, with which the inflection point, in this case, the transition from lumbar lordosis to thoracic kyphosis migrates cranially. On the other hand, the relationship between lumbar lordosis and pelvic incidence is also known, so both values should not differ by more than 10 degrees. With all this, the spines with a profile of lumbar lordosis and high pelvic incidence will be prone to the development of DS.

CLASSIFICATIONS

There are several classification systems, which we now introduce to the reader.

Wiltse classifies DS according to their anatomical/pathological origin (see Table 1). Marchetti and Bartolozzi in their 1990 classification differentiated spondylolisthesis from acquired or developmental origin. Their main contribution was to identify high-grade spondylolisthesis with certain specific characteristics, such as S1 endplate insufficiency, L5 trapezoidal index, verticality of the sacrum, and lumbosacral kyphosis (see Table 2). Then, Meyerding in this classification - which is the most frequently used-, spondylolisthesis is categorized by measuring the percentage of anterior displacement of the cranial vertebra over the caudal one. Grade I would correspond to a displacement between 0 and 25%, in grade II, the displacement would be between 26% and 50%, grade III corresponds between

51% and 75% and grade corresponds IV between 76% and 100%. Grade V would correspond to a displacement greater than 100%, or spondyloptosis. Finally, there is CARDS, specifically developed for degenerative spondylolisthesis. The CARDS classification system subdivides the broad spectrum of DS into reproducible subgroups [6], which would facilitate a common understanding among professionals dedicated to the investigation and treatment of this pathology. The classification assesses the height of the disc space, the sagittal alignment, and the translation of the listhesis segment and, in addition, it adds a modifier that is the presence of pain in the lower extremity (see Table **3**).

Table 1. Wiltse classification.

TYPE	DESCRIPTION
Dysplastic	Developmental defect of the sacrum or posterior arch of L5.
Isthmic	Pars interarticularis defect. A. Spondylolysis B. Elongation of the intact pars C. Pars fracture
Degenerative	Most frequent, located at L4-5.
Traumatic	Fracture localized elsewhere but the *Pars articularis*.
Pathological	Mainly caused by tumour or infection.

Table 2. Marchetti and Bartolozzi classification.

DEVELOPMENTAL	High grade dysplasia
	Low grade dysplasia
ACQUIRED	Traumatic
	Surgical
	Pathological
	Degenerative

Table 3. CARDS.

A TYPE	Advanced disc collapse without kyphosis. This collapse can be complete, placing the vertebral endplates parallel, or otherwise can be partial or even asymmetric, contacting the posterior portion of the vertebral bodies.
B TYPE	Disc partially preserved with translation less than 5 mm; no deformity in kyphosis.
C TYPE	Partially preserved disc with more than 5mm translation, but still without kyphosis.
D TYPE	Intervertebral kyphosis.
MODIFIER 0 **MODIFIER 1** **MODIFIER 2**	Without pain in the lower limbs Pain in one leg Pain in both legs

CLINICAL PRESENTATION

There are several epidemiological risk factors for the development of DS, as indicated above; female gender and age are among them, but the African-American ethnic group is also more prevalent than the white race [7]. Therefore, all these potential risk factors should be reflected in the clinical history.

The symptoms are similar to those of canal stenosis (within Arnoldi's classification, DS appears as an acquired subtype of degenerative origin). There is low back pain as the main symptom, which typically increases with extension and is frequent when going from sitting to standing. The pain radiates variably to one or both lower extremities, possibly causing either claudication with gait or radiculopathy. In the latter case, the most frequently affected root is L5, with pain appearing on the posterolateral aspect of the thigh, anterior tibia, and dorsum of the foot, with possible weakness for extension of the hallux.

DIAGNOSIS

In the anamnesis and clinical history, all the epidemiological factors must be collected, as well as the symptoms reported by the patient, differentiating the type of pain and its irradiation (differentiating between metameric and/or radicular).

In the physical examination, it is important to visualize the patient's position, as well as his way of walking or possible muscular atrophies. It can also guide the diagnosis of the "shape" of the spine, as well as the anatomical axes of the extremities and their mobility. The low back pain that the patient normally suffers can be reproduced or provoked by asking the patient to maintain an extension of the trunk in a standing position with the lower extremities in extension. A complete and directed neurological examination must be carried out, pointing out possible signs of root irritation, assessment of deep tendon reflexes, tactile discrimination, and muscle strength.

It is at the same time essential to identify other pathologies that can recreate similar symptoms; specially claudication of vascular origin (with its particular clinical peculiarities and in which it is possible to observe the absence of distal pulses) as well as pain radiating to the lower extremities of another origin, paying special attention to the exploration of the sacroiliac, hips and the abdominal region.

The definitive diagnosis, however, is made by means of imaging studies. It must be remembered that these studies should be carried out after a reasonable period of time from the onset of symptoms, as long as there is no response to conservative treatment, and in patients who do not present biological alarm signs, known as "red flags", such as affectation of the general condition, fever, obvious neurological signs (including cauda equina syndrome), *etc*. Plain radiography in lateral and anteroposterior projection in a standing position is the imaging test that is requested initially, in which we will typically observe the displacement of the vertebral body of L4 on L5. Sometimes it is difficult to determine if the observed listhesis is caused by lysis of the posterior arch or not, so it would be useful to request oblique projections when DS is suspected (fracture of the pars articularis is observed in lytic isthmic spondylolisthesis, known as Latarjet's puppy sign). Lateral dynamic radiographs in flexion and extension of the lumbar spine may also be useful, in which -following the accepted criteria (White, Panjabi, and Spector, modified by Vaccaro)- instability is diagnosed if there is a sagittal translation of more than 3.5 mm, or more than 15° of segmental kyphosis.On the other hand, subluxation, articular fracture or displacements may only be detected in dynamic radiographs.

Pre-surgical CT is useful for assessing bony structures, including subluxation, orientation, and/or tropism of the articular facets; and also provides information on the state of the pars articularis.

MRI is another study that is usually requested for the study of this pathology, it will give us information about the state of the soft tissues and those structures that may be involved in the symptoms. Both an effusion between the articular facets (the sign of possible instability) and hypertrophy of the ligamentum flavum or disc protrusions and adjacent disc degeneration can be observed, which may be the cause of central, lateral recess, and/or foraminal stenosis.

It should be taken into account that both the MRI and the CT study are performed in the supine position and normally, for the patient's comfort, with a pad under the knees. This positioning of the patient, which decreases lumbar lordosis, is important to be kept in mind because it can underdiagnose instability or displacement only detectable in dynamic studies.

From a diagnostic point of view as well as for the planning of surgical treatment, we believe it is essential to assess these patients with an anteroposterior and lateral teleradiography study of the entire spine in standing position, including the hips and skull. This test allows us to provide valuable information both for assessing the sagittal imbalance that causes the displacement of one vertebral body over another, as well as for the study of spinopelvic parameters and the possible recruitment by the patient of compensation measures in an attempt to achieve a rebalancing of the trunk, which take place in the rest of the spine, the pelvis and even the lower extremities.

Usually, an electromyographic study is also requested for neurological assessment, in which the most frequent root lesion can be observed, which is that of L5; nevertheless, this EMG does not replace a meticulous clinical examination and both must be interpreted together.

THE BODY'S REACTION: COMPENSATION MECHANISMS

Frequently many of these patients are in sagittal imbalance; it is well known that imbalances in this plane are correlated with poorer quality of life. Most of those who suffer from the disease present a non-physiological kyphosis in the L4-L5 segment. This alteration, added to the anterior displacement of the vertical sacral axis (SVA) due to the sliding of the L4 vertebral body, is the cause of the recruitment of compensation mechanisms [8]. The first compensation mechanisms to be activated are those of proximity to the lesion, that is, in the lumbar spine itself, which adopts a hyperlordosis in all the adjacent proximal lumbar segments, but especially in the L3-L4 segment. Similarly, the thoracic kyphosis is rectified by the contraction of the trunk extensor musculature in an attempt to rebalance the SVA, defined in the lateral radiography (Fig. **1**) as a radiological plumb line originating in the vertebral body of C7, and which should be -when the spine is balanced- passing through the posterosuperior border of L5-S1; if this plumb line falls in front, a positive value is given).

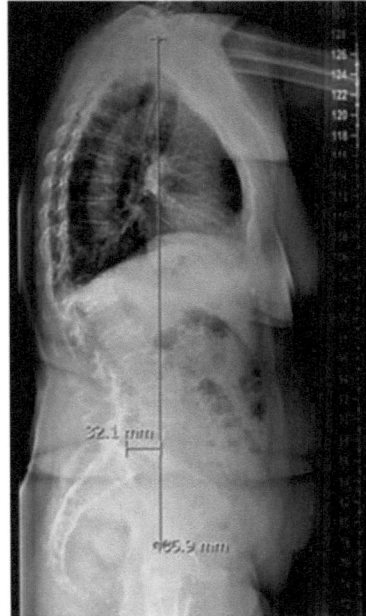

Fig. (1). SVA measurement (distance between the plumb line drawn from the center of the C7 vertebral body and the posterior angle of L5-S1) in a patient with degenerative spondylolisthesis.

These mechanisms require an increase in muscular work by the patient, which is quickly exhausted and causes part of the axial pain. If these are not effective or are insufficient to maintain balance, other compensation mechanisms are set in motion at the pelvic level, the latter adopting a retroversion disposition when rotating posteriorly on the coxofemoral joint.

Generally, these patients have high pelvic inclines [9], so they have a great capacity to achieve retroversion of the pelvis (reflected by the pelvic tilt parameter, also known as pelvic tilt-PT). If this backward rotation of the pelvis occurs and due to the almost absent mobility of the sacroiliac joints, a verticalization of the sacrum is caused by the consequent horizontalization of the upper plate of S1 (decreasing the value of the sacral inclination or slope -SS-), which also affects a posterior displacement of the patient's SVA, rebalancing the trunk.

Finally, if the compensation mechanisms of the spine and pelvis could not achieve balance, the lower extremities would be recruited secondarily to a greater pelvic retroversion through hip and knee flexion and ankle dorsiflexion. These joints must be explored, especially the hips, to rule out fixed deformities that require actions prior to or concomitant with those to be performed on the spine.

In our experience, we found that in patients undergoing surgery for DS, the most common spinopelvic and balance parameters were those of mild/moderate imbalance, generally with values of anterior displacement of the SVA of less than 5 cm, and that cannot be compensated by the hyperlordosis of the lumbar segments, which is increased -both in the values of lordosis in L3-L4 and T12-L4-, when compared with the general population. Therefore, compensation for the increase in lordosis in the proximal segments is activated, although DS patients continue to maintain a significant difference in the SVA value with respect to the control group. However, the values of distance to the SVA of the group of patients are less than 5cm, so they fall within the physiological range for the age group to which they belong and so that pelvic retroversion does not have to be activated to a great extent; it is true that the relative values of PT increase with respect to the control group, but these PT values all within the physiological range (<25°) and when they are put in context or related to their PI, which is also high and is compared with the relationship PT/PI of the control group, did not find significant differences between them.

In conclusion, this small SVA imbalance in ED patients is well tolerated and is not compensated for by the activation of the previously described pelvic retroversion mechanisms, probably because with proximal lumbar hyperlordosis

SVA values of less than 5 cm are obtained, which have slight clinical repercussions.

Let us analyze what we have just stated: Although it is true that there is a statistically significant difference in the values of pelvic tilt and pelvic incidence between populations with ED and the general population, it is equally true that these differences do not appear when comparing the percentage compensation between the two. This is a parameter that is defined by the quotient between the pelvic tilt and the pelvic incidence (PT/PI) and that we adapt as an index or indicator of the change in proportions on the basal state, so that it reflects the amount of pelvic tilt that it is recruited as a compensatory mechanism when we put it in relation to the pelvic incidence. The maximum theoretical compensation percentage is 100% and occurs when the pelvis is fully retroverted and the sacrum is fully vertical, this is so, because the pelvic incidence is the arithmetic sum of these two complementary angles, so if PI=PT+ SS and SS can be equal to 0, it turns out that PT=PI, recruiting 100% of the pelvic retroversion capacity determined by the pelvic incidence (Table **4**). This table shows that the percentage of compensation does not show significant differences between the populations, although these are between the absolute values of PT and PI as reflected in our study. Therefore, statistically higher PT values between both populations do not necessarily lead to the recruitment of pelvic retroversion.

Table 4. Compensation.

-	PT (°) P= 0,025	PI (°) P= 0,03	PT/PI (% compensation) NS
DS	18,8	60,45	31%
CONTROL	13,03	52,28	25%

That is, the compensation percentage is similar, they do not present statistically significant differences presenting similar percentage values. In other words, the population with ED has high PI and PT values in relation to the general population, but the relationship between the two when compared (PT/PI, defined as the percentage of compensation) does not differ between both populations, so that a high "absolute" PT value does not necessarily translate into pelvic retroversion.

The first and sometimes, in a high percentage of patients, the only compensation mechanisms that are activated are those of proximity to the lesion, in the lumbar spine itself.

In summary: in these patients with DD, both vertebral and pelvic compensation mechanisms were activated (in cases of greater imbalance) but, even so, they failed to return the spine to a state similar to that of the control population, maintaining a slight imbalance. Sagittal.

We believe that the latter is important when considering what type of surgical treatment should be performed. Among the most common surgical options that can be considered are: a) recalibration of the lumbar canal as a single gesture, b) arthrodesis with or without instrumentation, c) canal recalibration associated with arthrodesis, and d) canal recalibration and instrumented arthrodesis trying to correct the sagittal imbalance by means of osteotomies (for example, Ponte type) and correcting as much as possible both the slippage of L4 and the segmental kyphosis if present. The patient's comorbidities, imaging studies, and even the patient's age will help us when making this decision.

Currently, the debate on the need or not to fuse ED patients is in full swing and probably the criteria of dynamic stability and fragility should be the guide for the surgeon when planning the intervention of ED patients who are undergoing surgery. Surgical treatment has been indicated.

Is it necessary to intervene surgically in all DD patients, given that conceptually it is a situation of global instability of the spine, with a great concentration of stress in a single segment? Obviously not.

TREATMENT

The initial management of patients with ED should be conservative unless they present especially progressive motor neurological symptoms or sphincter incontinence. Conservative treatment is based on the medical treatment of pain and inflammation. NSAIDs should be administered in a short space of time and with gastroprotection, the same as corticosteroid treatment. We must bear in mind the incidence of comorbidities in this type of patient, who is already advanced in age on some occasions, especially smoking, diabetes, and, overall, frailty. The use of a lumbar belt and physical therapy can be effective in relieving the patient's symptoms. In the same way, the use of facet infiltrations and later its blocking by radiofrequency is frequent.

Messages to remember

1. The origin and development of ED are still unknown, probably multifactorial, although biomechanical factors play an important role.
2. Generally the symptoms are an association of lower back pain and canal stenosis, with gait claudication.

3. Dynamic radiographic studies are necessary to diagnose some patients.
4. When considering the indication for surgical treatment, the patient's sagittal profile must be taken into account.
5. For planning, the stability of the segment and the fragility of the patient must be evaluated.

CONCLUSION

The intrinsic instability of the olysthetic segment plays a key role in the fusion of such segments and in overall body balance. Compensatory mechanisms come into play both at the spine and at the pelvis (hips included, and then the knees).

REFERENCES

[1]   Lee JS, Suh KT, Kim JI, Lim JM, Goh TS. Association of estrogen receptor gene polymorphism in patients with degenerative lumbar spondylolisthesise. J Korean Neurosurg Soc 2011; 50(5): 415-9.
[http://dx.doi.org/10.3340/jkns.2011.50.5.415] [PMID: 22259687]

[2]   Abu-Leil S, Floman Y, Bronstein Y, Masharawi Y. A morphometric analysis of all lumbar intervertebral discs and vertebral bodies in degenerative spondylolisthesis. Eur Spine J 2016; 25(8): 2535-45.
[http://dx.doi.org/10.1007/s00586-016-4673-3] [PMID: 27349752]

[3]   Berlemann U, Jeszenszky DJ, Bühler DW, Harms J. The role of lumbar lordosis, vertebral end-plate inclination, disc height and facet orientation in degenerative spondylolisthesis Spinal Disord J. 1999; 12(1): 68-73.

[4]   Schuller S, Charles YP, Steib JP. Sagittal spinopelvic alignment and body mass index in patients with degenerative spondylolisthesis. Eur Spine J 2011; 20(5): 713-9.
[http://dx.doi.org/10.1007/s00586-010-1640-2] [PMID: 21116661]

[5]   Roussouly P, Pinheiro-Franco JL. Biomechanical analysis of the spino-pelvic organization and adaptation in pathology. Eur Spine J 2011; 20(S5) (Suppl. 5): 609-18.
[http://dx.doi.org/10.1007/s00586-011-1928-x] [PMID: 21809016]

[6]   Kepler CK, Hilibrand AS, Sayadipour A, *et al.* Clinical and radiographic degenerative spondylolisthesis (CARDS) classification. Spine J 2015; 15(8): 1804-11.
[http://dx.doi.org/10.1016/j.spinee.2014.03.045] [PMID: 24704503]

[7]   Vogt MT, Rubin DA, Palermo L, *et al.* Lumbar spine listhesis in older African American women. Spine J 2003; 3(4): 255-61.
[http://dx.doi.org/10.1016/S1529-9430(03)00024-X] [PMID: 14589183]

[8]   Gille O, Challier V, Parent H, *et al.* Degenerative lumbar spondylolisthesis. Cohort of 670 patients, and proposal of a new classification. Orthop Traumatol Surg Res 2014; 100(6) (Suppl.): S311-5.
[http://dx.doi.org/10.1016/j.otsr.2014.07.006] [PMID: 25201282]

[9]   Funao H, Tsuji T, Hosogane N, *et al.* Comparative study of spinopelvic sagittal alignment between patients with and without degenerative spondylolisthesis. Eur Spine J 2012; 21(11): 2181-7.
[http://dx.doi.org/10.1007/s00586-012-2374-0] [PMID: 22639298]

CHAPTER 6

Biomechanics of Interspinous Devices: The Option to Stabilize without Fusion

Parchi Paolo Domenico[1,*] and **Javier Melchor Duart-Clemente**[2]

[1] *1st Orthopedic and Traumatology Division, Department of translational research and new technology in medicine and surgery, University of Pisa, Pisa, Italy*

[2] *Neurosurgery and Spinal Surgery Departments, Valencia General Hospital, Valencia, Spain*

Abstract: Several interspinous devices have been incorporated into the spinal implant market. There have been several reasons for their wide use, including that they can be implanted using a minimally invasive approach even under local anesthesia. This chapter reviews the biomechanical studies about interspinous devices to allow the reader a better comprehension of the effects of these devices, not only on the treated segment but also on the adjacent segments of the spine. Unfortunately, the use of these implants is often not associated with a thorough understanding of their biomechanical behaviour, which is useful to address both indications and contraindications for this procedure.

Keywords: Dynamic spinal stabilization, Interspinous devices, Motion preservation devices.

INTRODUCTION

Interspinous devices (ISD) are implants that are inserted between the spinous processes of two neighboring vertebrae in order to maintain distraction. These devices are constructed using various materials, including titanium, polyetheretherketone (PEEK), and elastomeric compounds [1]. Initially, ISD implantation was primarily indicated for lumbar stenosis, especially in cases where symptoms improved with flexion. However, its applications have expanded to include other surgical indications, such as grade I degenerative spondylolisthesis, discogenic low back pain, non-traumatic instability, and facet syndrome [2, 3]. It is important to note that ISDs do not play a role in preventing disc reherniation. Additionally, these devices are utilized to prevent adjacent segment disease. Even in the surgical treatment of occupational low back pain, the

* **Corresponding author Parchi Paolo Domenico:** 1st Orthopedic and Traumatology Division, Department of translational research and new technology in medicine and surgery, University of Pisa, Pisa, Italy; E-mail: paolo.parchi@unipi.it

Javier Melchor Duart Clemente (Ed.)

use of interspinous spacers offers advantages such as reduced invasiveness and morbidity, increased range of motion, decreased overload on adjacent levels, comparable clinical outcomes, and improved work results when compared to arthrodesis.

These devices have been created with the purpose of opening the spinal canal, restoring foraminal height, and relieving pressure on the facet joints. They offer sufficient stability, particularly during extension, while still allowing movement in the treated area [4]. By preserving the range of motion in the implanted segment, these devices prevent or minimize the risk of overloading and premature degeneration in the adjacent segments, which is in contrast to the effects of fusion [5]. In addition to these motion-preserving devices, another type of interspinous device has been developed to promote the fusion of the interspinous space [6], as explained further below.

This chapter provides an overview of the biomechanical research conducted on interspinous devices, aiming to enhance the reader's understanding of the impact of these devices. It not only focuses on the treated segment but also examines the influence on the neighboring segments of the spine. Regrettably, the utilization of these implants frequently occurs without a comprehensive comprehension of their biomechanical characteristics, which is crucial for determining the appropriate indications and contraindications for this procedure.

CLASSIFICATION OF INTERSPINOUS DEVICES

The interspinous devices currently in the market could be classified into two main groups: motion preservation devices and devices that fuse the interspinous space.

Motion Preservation Devices

These were the initial interspinous devices developed for the treatment of spinal stenosis, by blocking extension, which in turn can be achieved either in a rigid or a flexible manner. The former –also called static- devices consist of non-compressible materials of different biomechanical properties with the same mechanism of action, providing a wedge between the spinous processes causing a fixed distraction during extension. On the other hand, flexible or dynamic devices –which are different due to their material and/or to their shape- offer a higher level of elasticity that allows their deformation during extension of the segment in which they have been implanted, acting as a rear shock absorber. While rigid devices may be compared to a stone preventing a door from opening, flexible devices may be compared to a rubber stopper.

Fusion Devices

These kinds of devices merged as an evolution of the mobile ones in order to overcome their lack of stability in axial rotation; they may have paired plates with teeth or maybe U-shaped devices with wings that are attached to the spinous process. They are supposed, when used with interbody fusion, to be an alternative to pedicle screws -rod constructs to aid in the stabilization of the spine, being less invasive and with fewer risks than pedicle (or facet) screws.

BIOMECHANICAL EFFECTS OF INTERSPINOUS DEVICES

Biomechanics Effects of Nonfusion Interspinous Devices

From the review of the studies on the biomechanics of non-fusion interspinous devices available in the literature, we have focused our attention on the analysis of the following biomechanical effects:

1. Influence on the range of movement (ROM) of the treated segment and of the adjacent segments;
2. Influence on the size of the spinal canal area and foraminal canal area;
3. Effects on the intradiscal pressure, disc load, and facet load;
4. Influence on the segmental tilt and instantaneous axis of rotation (IAR) of the treated segment.

Influence on the Range of Movement (ROM) of the Treated Segment and the Adjacent Segments

New interspinous devices have undergone testing and comparison to determine if their implantation affects the movement characteristics of the involved vertebrae in different clinical scenarios, such as intact and destabilized conditions. The impact of these devices on not only the instrumented level but also the adjacent levels has been extensively studied using cadaveric specimens and Finite Element Modelling. In a study by Lindsey [7], the X-Stop device was found to only reduce the range of motion (ROM) in flexion-extension at the implanted levels, without affecting the other vertebral functional units, despite a slight decrease in lordosis (2°). However, when considering decompressive procedures commonly performed in spinal surgeries, the biomechanical outcomes may vary. Phillips [8] investigated the effect of partial facetectomy and discectomy and found that the insertion of a different interspinous spacer, the DIAM device, improved certain values after destabilization caused by discectomy. Although the DIAM device restored postdiscectomy motion in flexion extension to levels below intact values, it did not have the same effect on other movement modalities. In lateral bending, it reduced the increased motion caused by discectomy but not enough to reach the intact segment level. Additionally, it did not reduce the increased axial rotation induced by discectomy, resulting in a motion larger than the intact value.

In a biomechanical *in vitro* study, the Coflex device's stabilization effect was evaluated in partially and completely destabilized segments, and compared to the use of a pedicle screw [9]. Surprisingly, the results for flexion/extension and axial rotation indicate that the Coflex device could be beneficial clinically in both planes, not just one. It permits motion significantly less than that in the destabilized specimens and is comparable to intact specimens. The findings in both flexion/extension and axial rotation demonstrate that the device provides non-rigid fixation and can restore normal motion characteristics in these two planes for destabilized specimens. Another study on the same device [10] conducted a finite element analysis by applying mechanical loads based on postural changes. The study revealed that Coflex significantly limited L4/L5 displacement in extension (24.5%) and lateral bending (44.5%) compared to a control group, with flexion being minimally reduced by 1.3%. The authors also noted intense stress (120 MPa) on the base of the spinous process during extension, which could explain the common occurrence of spinous process fractures during follow-up, especially when used in 2 adjacent levels due to the sandwich phenomenon. This may also be related to the fact that this is the only ISP that increases both disc and facet joint stresses in the distal adjacent segment [11].

A combination of both study methods was utilized in the Lafage study: an *in vitro* and finite-element analysis were combined to evaluate the biomechanical impact of the Wallis device on a vertebral segment [12]. The study compared intact segments, injured segments, and instrumented segments (L4-L5) under various loads in flexionextension, lateral bending, and torsion. The implant's effect was most noticeable in flexion extension, with experimental results showing a reduced range of motion in the instrumented spine compared to the injured and intact ones. Additionally, finite-element analysis indicated a decrease in disc stresses and an increase in loads transmitted to the spinous processes. Another cadaveric study on the same interspinous device demonstrated that the Wallis device reduced flexion extension at L3-4 by 13.8% but increased lateral bending and axial rotation range of motion by 6.2% and 0.4%, respectively [13].

Besides individual analyses of these devices, there have been comparisons made among them. Wilke conducted an *in vitro* study to evaluate the biomechanical impact of four different interspinous implants (Coflex, Wallis, DIAM, and X-Stop) [4] on human lumbar spine specimens divided into four equal groups and subjected to pure moments in flexion/extension, lateral bending, and axial rotation: 1/ intact, 2/ defect, and 3/ after implantation. Both the range of motion and intradiscal pressure were measured. Generally, the defect led to an increase in ROM compared to the intact state in all loading directions, and none of these interspinous devices could fully counteract this destabilizing effect in any of the three loading directions, except for extension. Only the Wallis device showed a tendency to stabilize the specimens to the levels of the intact ones in flexion (due to its strings that limit flexion by wrapping around adjacent spinous devices). In terms of the other two directions, lateral bending allowed slightly more motion with these implants compared to the intact state, while for axial rotation, the implants were unable to compensate for the destabilization caused by the defect. However, other research indicates that the DIAM appears to replicate the biomechanical properties of the intact lumbar spine more accurately than other interspinous devices, particularly in terms of Range of Movement [14].

Following the introduction of percutaneous interspinous devices, several studies have been conducted to determine their efficacy compared to previous devices. One such study focused on the In-Space implant, which can be implanted percutaneously, and evaluated its impact on the range of motion (ROM) and intervertebral disc pressure (DP) at the implanted level and adjacent levels [13]. The study found that the extension ROM at the implanted level, with or without discectomy, was significantly reduced in both cases. However, this reduction was compensated by an increase in ROM at the adjacent levels. No significant changes in ROM were observed in any other modes of motion or at any other levels studied. The authors concluded that the In-Space interspinous spacer effectively stabilizes the spine and reduces intervertebral disc pressure at the instrumented level during extension, without significant effects on the adjacent segment.

Once again, a comparison was conducted among various interspinous devices, both those implanted with traditional open surgery and those implanted percutaneously. A biomechanical evaluation was performed in a laboratory setting to assess the changes in a range of motion in the affected and adjacent segments after the implantation of four different interspinous devices: Aperius, In-Space, X-Stop, and Coflex (the first two being percutaneous). The focus of this study was to evaluate the impact of preload conditions on the range of motion of the lumbar spine when implanted with these devices. All interspinous devices resulted in a significant reduction in the range of motion during extension at the instrumented segment, without significantly affecting other directions of motion, both with and without the application of preload. The range of motion during flexion was reduced by all implants only when preload was applied. However, despite this, all tested devices exhibited an increase in the range of motion of the adjacent segment. It could be speculated that this may lead to an increased risk of adjacent segment degeneration, but this risk should also be balanced against the risks associated with the operated and destabilized operative level.

Influence on the Size of the Spinal Canal Area (SCA) and Foraminal Canals Area (FCA)

Considering that the initial and primary clinical indication for implanting these devices was the neurogenic claudication caused by spinal stenosis with improvement with flexion, it is important to note that a combination of mechanical and vascular factors has been suggested to explain neurogenic claudication. However, the mechanical factor may be the main one, as patients experience improvement with flexion. This is because in this position the spinal canal opens up, relieving compression and vascular insult to the lumbar roots. This is why these devices gained popularity, as they place the spine in a flexed position by limiting extension, resulting in less invasive surgery compared to open decompressive surgery. This is particularly beneficial for elderly patients and can even be performed on an outpatient basis under local anesthesia. Now, let's delve into the biomechanical basis for this phenomenon.

Several research studies have examined the impact of the initial interspinous X-Stop interspinous spacer on the dimensions of the spinal canal and neural foramina during flexion and extension *in vitro* using cadaveric specimens, comparing intact and implanted specimens. The most significant increase was observed in the subarticular diameter (50%), foraminal width (41%), and area (25%) -with a 17% increase in patients who were implanted with Aperius PercLID for *claudicatio spinalis*, one of the earliest percutaneous interspinous devices to be introduced. Additionally, there was an increase in the canal area (18%) and diameter (10%). These findings demonstrate that the implant helps prevent the narrowing of the spinal canal and neural foramina during extension. In fact, a recent study [15] with Aperius revealed with axial loading MRI that, although there was no significant increase in the dural sac cross-sectional areas at the operated level, it did prevent the decrease observed in adjacent levels. Another study conducted *in vivo* using the same implant found that the cross-sectional foraminal area at the implanted level increased by 36.5% with the X-Stop device in ten elderly lumbar spinal stenosis patients. Additionally, there was a mean expansion of the spinal canal by 22%, showing significant differences between standing, seated neutral, and seated extended positions. This trend was also observed in several level diseases, where positional MRI indicated enlargement of the foraminal area in extension at a single diseased level (with at least a 20% increase) in elderly lumbar spinal stenosis patients [16]. Another aspect of the study measured the vertical and horizontal shortest distances in the interspinous space at the implanted and adjacent segments during weight-bearing functional activities both before and after implantation of the device. The results showed an increase of one-third and one-fourth in the foraminal area and width, respectively, during extension, while minimal changes were observed in standing and flexion positions. This suggests an effective distraction of the interspinous space *in vivo* without causing significant kinematic disturbances at the adjacent segments.

Effects on the Intradiscal Pressure and Facet Load

In addition to the impact on the ROM and the opening of the spinal foramina, it is important to determine the potential influence of these interspinous devices on the disc and facet pressures. Numerous studies have been conducted to investigate this matter.

Swanson conducted a study [17] on the pressure of cadaveric discs after the insertion of an X-stop device of an appropriate size. The study utilized a pressure transducer to measure the intradiscal pressure and annular stresses in various positions such as flexion, neutral, and extension. The authors observed a decrease in pressures in the posterior *annulus* and *nucleus pulposus* by one-third and two-fifths, respectively in the neutral and standing positions. This reduction was even greater in the extension position. Similarly, another study by Wilke compared different interspinous devices including Coflex, Wallis, DIAM, and X-Stop. In all four implant groups, the intradiscal pressure was significantly reduced during extension. However, none of the implants caused a significant change in intradiscal pressure during flexion, lateral bending, and axial rotation. This finding was consistent with the In-Space device, which only achieved a reduction in intradiscal pressure at L3-4 during extension.

Another study regarding biomechanics was recently published [18], focusing on the impact of varying degrees of distraction of interspinous processes on the distribution of pressure within the lumbar intervertebral disc. The researchers posited that different levels of distraction following the placement of an interspinous device would lead to distinct alterations in disc pressure distribution at the instrumentation level. The most effective implant would be one that could significantly reduce pressure within the posterior *annulus* and *nucleus*, while diverting a substantial portion of the load away from the intervertebral disc towards the spinous processes in extension and neutral positions, without causing any significant changes in load distribution in other areas of the disc at the instrumented level. The study revealed a direct relationship between the height of the spacer and load sharing. Specifically, an interspinous device with a spacer height equivalent to the interspinous process distance in the neutral position was able to effectively distribute biomechanical disc load without causing a significant shift in load within the anterior *annulus*, with approximately half of the load in the posterior *annulus* being shared by the implant during extension. Conversely, when an interspinous device with a spacer height greater than the interspinous process distance in the neutral position was used, there was a significant increase in load within the anterior *annulus* by approximately 400%, despite effective load sharing in extension, neutral, and flexion positions within the posterior *annulus*. This increase in anterior *annulus* load could potentially accelerate disc degeneration, at least in theory. Interspinous devices function as a pivot point in segmental motion, redirecting force from the posterior *annulus* to the spinous process; the extent of interspinous process distraction caused by this pivot point is directly linked to load distribution on the intervertebral disc. More recently, interlaminar devices have been developed as an enhancement of interspinous devices, offering benefits such as increased segmental stability, reduced disc stress as well as reduced risk of spinous process fracture and thus device failure globally [19].

Conversely, Wiseman *et al.* examined the facet loading parameters of lumbar cadaver spines in extension both before and after the insertion of an X-Stop [20]. They discovered that, at the level of the implant, there was a significant decrease in mean peak and average pressure, contact area, and force, with no significant changes at adjacent levels, except for contact area at the level above the implant, which could potentially lead to facet pain or accelerated facet joint degeneration. In a similar vein, the placement of the In-Space interspinous device reduced mean facet load by one-third during flexion and two-thirds during extension in an *in vitro* biomechanical study using nondestructive cadaveric flexibility testing conducted by Lazaro [21]. This reduction was accompanied by the expected significant decrease in range of motion during extension, and a less significant reduction in foraminal height during extension compared to the normal state.

Influence on the Segmental Tilt and Instantaneous Axis of Rotation (IAR) of the Treated Segment

As local and global alignment has become an essential issue regarding spinal procedures in order to improve clinical results, this also applies to the implantation of interspinous devices.

In Wilke's study [4], a very minor kyphotic deformation of 0.6 degrees was observed in human specimens after surgical decompression. Among all interspinous devices tested, only the DIAM had a minimal increasing effect on this deformation. This particular finding was also confirmed in a biomechanical study using a lumbar porcine model by Anasetti [22], which demonstrated a posterior shift of the IAR. Interestingly, the use of laces -which are attached to the adjacent spinous processes- of the DIAM can limit flexion and keep the IAR aligned with the intact spine at the center of the disc. Conversely, oversizing the implant was found to restrict movements more significantly, potentially leading to a flexed position of the segment. Fortunately, it appears that ISD does not impact sagittal balance [23], as any initial loss of local lordosis may be temporary, with the intervertebral space realigning spontaneously during mid-term follow-up [24].

Zheng *et al.* [18] have also conducted research on the matter of choosing the appropriate height for the device. They experimented with various sizes of the same interspinous implant. On one hand, increasing the size of the implant leads to a greater expansion of the *canal* and *foramina* diameters, which is beneficial for treating stenosis. However, this also results in more kyphosis and load on the anterior disc, potentially causing disc degeneration (Fig. 1). On the other hand, if the height of the implant is only equal to the distance between the interspinous processes, the canal opening may not be as effective and may not sufficiently improve symptomatic stenosis.

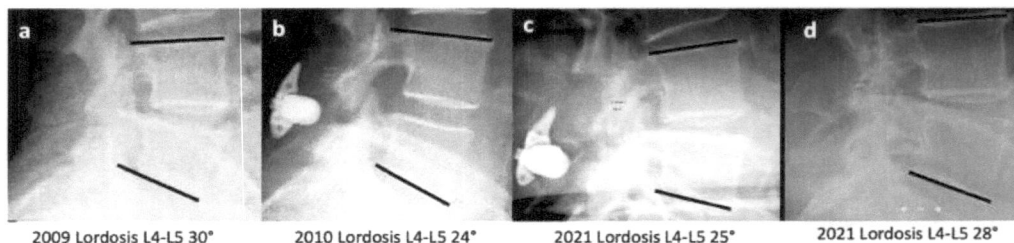

| 2009 Lordosis L4-L5 30° | 2010 Lordosis L4-L5 24° | 2021 Lordosis L4-L5 25° | 2021 Lordosis L4-L5 28° |

Fig. (1). Segmentary L4-L5 kyphosis after the implantation of a stand-alone X-STOP interspinous device (**a**) L4-L5 sagittal balance before the X-Stop implantation: L4-L5 lordosis 30°. (**b**) L4-L5 Sagittal balance after 1 year from the X-Stop device implantation: L4-L5 lordosis 24°. (**c**) L4-L5 Sagittal balance after 11 years from the X-Stop device implantation: L4-L5 lordosis 25°. (**d**) L4-L5 Sagittal balance after the X-Stop device removal for intense lumbar pain: L4-L5 lordosis 28°.

Biomechanics Effects of Fusion Interspinous Devices

The interspinous devices were originally created to provide both stabilization and motion preservation. However, a new design was developed to achieve stabilization in lateral flexion or rotation, resulting in the introduction of fixed interspinous devices as an alternative to pedicle screw fixation for fusion. The market introduction of fusion interspinous devices is relatively recent, leading to fewer studies on the biomechanical effects of these devices, particularly focusing on the reduction of range of motion compared to pedicle screw constructs.

The concept of a fixed interspinous device was conceived during a study conducted by Kettler *et al.* to enhance biomechanical performance in terms of improved stabilization. The study [25] focused on a modified version of the Coflex interspinous implant, known as Coflex Rivet (now Coflex F -for fusion-), which involved screw-fixation to the spinous processes. Unlike the original version, this variation successfully addressed the destabilizing effects of surgical defects in axial rotation and lateral bending, while also providing stabilization in flexion (excluding extension). This development opened up new possibilities for the application of such devices. However, a drawback of interspinous fusion devices is the increase in range of motion (ROM) at adjacent segments, particularly in flexion extension. This is believed to be a compensatory mechanism due to heightened stiffness at the instrumented level [26].

In addition to the Coflex F, which serves as a genuine interspinous fusion device, there are other fixed "interspinous" devices that have adopted different designs, primarily involving spinous transfixion. Some of these devices have undergone development and testing in comparison to pedicle screw fixation. The results have shown that they possess a stabilizing effect similar to pedicle screw fixation, but only in flexion extension. For instance, the CD HORIZON SPIRE (Wang [27]) together with various studies on the ASPEN device, in conjunction with different interbody fusions like ALIF (Karahalios [28]) and TLIF (Kaibara [29], Techy [30]), have demonstrated limitations in range of motion solely in flexion-extension, comparable to a bilateral pedicle screw construct. However, these devices do not significantly impact lateral bending or axial rotation. Interestingly, a similar study involving expandable PLIF cages also exhibited stabilization in axial rotation (Gonzalez-Blohm [31]).

DISCUSSION

As previously mentioned, ISD has emerged as an alternative treatment for spinal stenosis. When compared to other surgical options such as open decompression surgery or fusion for symptomatic lumbar stenosis, ISD has been shown to have fewer complications and long-term costs when used as the initial surgical treatment [32]. Although reoperation may be required, the addition of ISD to traditional open decompressive surgery has resulted in better clinical outcomes. This includes improvements in VAS back pain and radiological parameters such as foraminal height and disc height at the posterior part [33]. Furthermore, ISD has demonstrated superior improvement in VAS back pain compared to endoscopy [34].

The initial clinical indication for ISD was spinal stenosis causing neurogenic claudication. However, it can also assist in unloading facets or discs, whether degenerated or not, at the index level or above, adjacent to it. This is done in order to prevent Adjacent Segment Disease (ASD), also known as "topping-off". In comparison to rigid fixation, ISD is more similar to the intact lumbar spine in terms of Range of Movement, Intradiscal Pressure, and facet joint forces. These similarities could potentially reduce the occurrence of adjacent segment degeneration in the long run [35]. The DIAM system, with its biomechanical characteristics [36], maybe the preferred choice for this indication due to its better performance compared to pedicle-based dynamic systems [37]. Additionally, the DIAM system has shown lower ROM at adjacent levels [38], although intradiscal pressure may slightly increase in cases used for ASD prevention after circumferential fusion [39]. Even when considering the instrumentation of 2 adjacent levels, the DIAM implant could provide protection too. However, it is important to note that compensation for the lack of movement due to ISD stabilization could potentially increase ROM and promote ASD [40].

As previously elucidated, from a biomechanical standpoint, the various interspinous (nonfusion) devices enhance stability in extension but do not address instability in axial rotation, lateral bending, and occasionally in flexion [1, 3, 6]; by placing this device between the spinous processes, not only is there a distraction between them, but there is also an enlargement of the spinal and foraminal canals, all without significantly overburdening adjacent segments [1, 24]. The inserted device functions as a pivot during extension movements, leading to a posterior shift of the IAR and providing relief to the facet joints and posterior *annulus fibrosus* [10].

It is crucial to attain an appropriate level of distraction, sufficient to stabilize the segment but not excessive to the point of overdistraction. This is because inducing a kyphotic position could lead to disc overloading and premature degeneration. Therefore, the selection of the current implant size appears to play a significant role in the patient's clinical outcome, providing relief from pain in individuals with lumbar spinal stenosis and preventing anterior disc degeneration. In order to achieve accurate implantation and avoid overestimating the device size, some authors suggest measuring the distance between the spinous processes or utilizing device templates, if available, instead of relying solely on the operating positions, which may induce excessive spinal flexion.

It is important to bear in mind the potential for causing a segmental kyphosis in the lumbar spine, which is normally lordotic. This can lead to excessive stress on the intervertebral disc, resulting in premature degeneration (Fig. **2**) [40]. The introduction of ISD has filled the gaps in indications that were previously unaddressed. However, it is essential to provide accurate indications to ensure favorable clinical outcomes and minimize the risk of excessive failures.

Interspinous distraction may improve clinical stenosis -irrespective of their design-, having an immediately measurable neurophysiological effect as that achieved after surgical release [41]. Nevertheless, implantation of these devices is not free of complications, and adverse effects could occur, such as spinous process fracture, device migration (which can be solved even percutaneously in those cases of the percutaneous approach [42]), as well as pain or symptoms relapse [43]. We have to bear in mind that IPD may not be suitable for some indications which may require more sound stabilization -such as pedicle screw fusion-, that remains the gold standard in most surgical procedures in which the goal is a stable arthrodesis; it must not be forgotten than surgical treatments for spinal conditions should be best indicated and performed by neurosurgeons or spine surgeons [44]. During the implantation of the interspinous device, great attention should be paid to bone quality and proper distraction -avoiding excessive ones which could favour complications [45]-, as well as anatomical characteristics of the spinous process [46]. Anyhow, the evolution of the design of these devices decreases both device complications and reoperations, which are fewer with the next generation of interspinous devices [47].

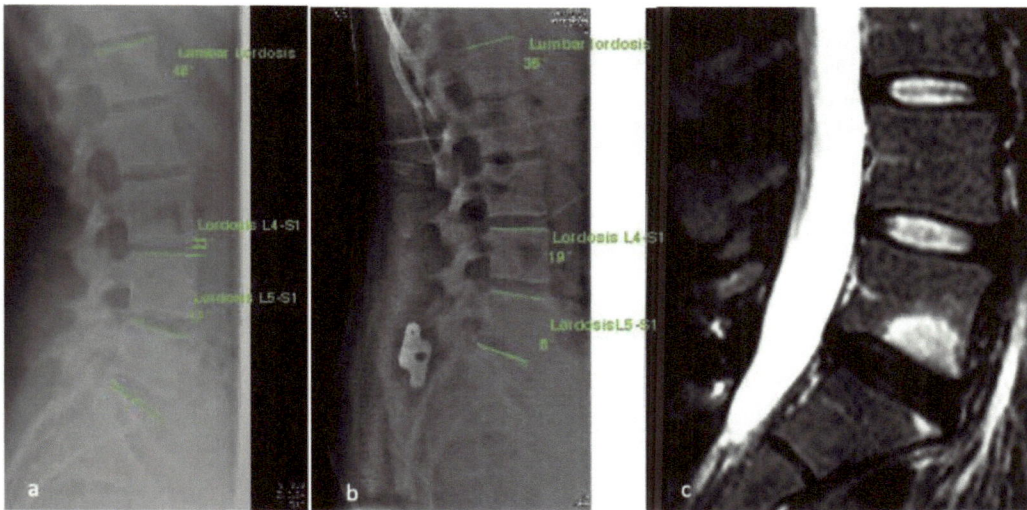

Fig. (2). Segmentary L5-S1 kyphosis after the implantation of a stand-alone ASPEN interspinous device with overload of the anterior part of the intervertebral disc. (**a**) Sagittal balance of lumbar spine before the implantation of the ASPEN device lumbar lordosis 48°, L4-S1 lordosis 33°, and L5-S1 lordosis 17° . (**b**) Sagittal balance of lumbar spine after 4 years from the ASPEN device implantation: lumbar lordosis 35°, L4-S1 lordosis 19°, and L5-S1 lordosis 8°. (**c**) MRI scan after 4 years from the Aspen implantation that shows anterior disc endplate degeneration.

CONCLUSION

Not all the interspinous devices are the same nor behave biomechanically in the same way. It is important to understand the benefits and risks of these, in order to choose the proper one for a particular patient depending on the indication and the clinical characteristics of the patient.

REFERENCES

[1]   Bono CM, Vaccaro AR. Interspinous process devices in the lumbar spine. J Spinal Disord Tech 2007; 20(3): 255-61.
[http://dx.doi.org/10.1097/BSD.0b013e3180331352] [PMID: 17473649]

[2]   Kabir SMR, Gupta SR, Casey ATH. Lumbar interspinous spacers: a systematic review of clinical and biomechanical evidence. Spine 2010; 35(25): E1499-506.
[http://dx.doi.org/10.1097/BRS.0b013e3181e9af93] [PMID: 21102279]

[3]   Gazzeri R, Galarza M, Alfieri A. Controversies about interspinous process devices in the treatment of degenerative lumbar spine diseases: past, present, and future. BioMed Research International 2014; 1-15. 975052.
[http://dx.doi.org/10.1155/2014/975052]

[4]   Wilke HJ, Drumm J, Häussler K, Mack C, Steudel WI, Kettler A. Biomechanical effect of different lumbar interspinous implants on flexibility and intradiscal pressure. Eur Spine J 2008; 17(8): 1049-56.
[http://dx.doi.org/10.1007/s00586-008-0657-2] [PMID: 18584219]

[5]   Richards JC, Majumdar S, Lindsey DP, Beaupré GS, Yerby SA. The treatment mechanism of an interspinous process implant for lumbar neurogenic intermittent claudication. Spine 2005; 30(7): 744-9.
[http://dx.doi.org/10.1097/01.brs.0000157483.28505.e3] [PMID: 15803075]

[6]   Wu JC, Mummaneni PV. Using lumbar interspinous anchor with transforaminal lumbar interbody fixation. World Neurosurg 2010; 73(5): 471-2.
[http://dx.doi.org/10.1016/j.wneu.2010.03.005] [PMID: 20920928]

[7]   Lindsey DP, Swanson KE, Fuchs P, Hsu KY, Zucherman JF, Yerby SA. The effects of an interspinous implant on the kinematics of the instrumented and adjacent levels in the lumbar spine. Spine 203; 28, 19, 2192–2197.
[http://dx.doi.org/10.1097/01.BRS.0000084877.88192.8E]

[8]   Phillips FM, Voronov LI, Gaitanis IN, Carandang G, Havey RM, Patwardhan AG. Biomechanics of posterior dynamic stabilizing device (DIAM) after facetectomy and discectomy. Spine J 2006; 6(6): 714-22.
[http://dx.doi.org/10.1016/j.spinee.2006.02.003] [PMID: 17088203]

[9]   Tsai KJ, Murakami H, Lowery GL, Hutton WC. A biomechanical evaluation of an interspinous device (Coflex) used to stabilize the lumbar spine. J Surg Orthop Adv 2006; 15(3): 167-72.
[PMID: 17087886]

[10]   Byun DH, Shin DA, Kim JM, Kim SH, Kim HI. Finite element analysis of the biomechanical effect of coflex™ on the lumbar spine. Korean J Spine 2012; 9(3): 131-6.
[http://dx.doi.org/10.14245/kjs.2012.9.3.131] [PMID: 25983803]

[11]   Liu Z, Zhang S, Li J, Tang H. Biomechanical comparison of different interspinous process devices in the treatment of lumbar spinal stenosis: a finite element analysis. BMC Musculoskelet Disord 2022; 17;23(1): 585.
[http://dx.doi.org/10.1186/s12891-022-05543-y]

[12]   Lafage V, Gangnet N, Sénégas J, Lavaste F, Skalli W. New interspinous implant evaluation using an *in vitro* biomechanical study combined with a finite-element analysis. Spine 2007; 32(16): 1706-13.
[http://dx.doi.org/10.1097/BRS.0b013e3180b9f429] [PMID: 17632390]

[13]   Ilharreborde B, Shaw MN, Berglund LJ, Zhao KD, Gay RE, An KN. Biomechanical evaluation of posterior lumbar dynamic stabilization: an *in vitro* comparison between Universal Clamp and Wallis systems. Eur Spine J 2011; 20(2): 289-96.
[http://dx.doi.org/10.1007/s00586-010-1641-1] [PMID: 21132335]

[14]   Shen H, Fogel GR, Zhu J, Liao Z, Liu W. Biomechanical analysis of different lumbar interspinous process devices: a finite element study. World Neurosurg 2019; 127: e1112-9.

[http://dx.doi.org/10.1016/j.wneu.2019.04.051] [PMID: 30980982]

[15]   Hjaltadottir H, Hebelka H, Molinder C, Brisby H, Baranto A. Axial loading during MRI reveals insufficient effect of percutaneous interspinous implants (Aperius™ PerCLID™) on spinal canal area. Eur Spine J 2020; 29(1): 122-8.
[http://dx.doi.org/10.1007/s00586-019-06159-y] [PMID: 31584119]

[16]   Siddiqui M, Karadimas E, Nicol M, Smith FW, Wardlaw D. Influence of X Stop on neural foramina and spinal canal area in spinal stenosis. Spine 2006; 31(25): 2958-62.
[http://dx.doi.org/10.1097/01.brs.0000247797.92847.7d] [PMID: 17139227]

[17]   Swanson KE, Lindsey DP, Hsu KY, Zucherman JF, Yerby SA. The effects of an interspinous implant on intervertebral disc pressures. Spine 2003; 28(1): 26-32.
[http://dx.doi.org/10.1097/00007632-200301010-00008] [PMID: 12544951]

[18]   Zheng S, Yao Q, Cheng L, *et al.* The effects of a new shape-memory alloy interspinous process device on the distribution of intervertebral disc pressures *in vitro*. J Biomed Res 2010; 24(2): 115-23.
[http://dx.doi.org/10.1016/S1674-8301(10)60019-X] [PMID: 23554621]

[19]   Lu T, Lu Y. Interlaminar stabilization offers greater biomechanical advantage compared to interspinous stabilization after lumbar decompression: a finite element analysis. J Orthop Surg Res 2020; 15(1): 291.
[http://dx.doi.org/10.1186/s13018-020-01812-5] [PMID: 32727615]

[20]   Wiseman CM, Lindsey DP, Fredrick AD, Yerby SA. The effect of an interspinous process implant on facet loading during extension. Spine 2005; 30(8): 903-7.
[http://dx.doi.org/10.1097/01.brs.0000158876.51771.f8] [PMID: 15834334]

[21]   Lazaro BC, Brasiliense LB, Sawa AG, *et al.* Biomechanics of a novel minimally invasive lumbar interspinous spacer: effects on kinematics, facet loads, and foramen height. Neurosurgery 2010; 66(3) (Suppl Operative): 126-32.
[PMID: 20173562]

[22]   Anasetti F, Galbusera F, Aziz HN, *et al.* Spine stability after implantation of an interspinous device: an *in vitro* and finite element biomechanical study. J Neurosurg Spine 2010; 13(5): 568-75.
[http://dx.doi.org/10.3171/2010.6.SPINE09885] [PMID: 21039145]

[23]   Bistazzoni S, Angelis MD, ercole MD, *et al.* Evaluation of effect of posterior dynamic stabilization intraspin system on sagittal spinal balance using EOS® X-ray imaging system. J Neurol Neurophysiol 2017; 8(4): 4.
[http://dx.doi.org/10.4172/2155-9562.1000439]

[24]   Wang DF, *et al.* The effect of interlaminar Coflex stabilization in the topping-off procedure on local and global spinal sagittal alignment. BMC Musculoskelet Disord 2023; 11;24(1): 116.
[http://dx.doi.org/10.1186/s12891-023-06231-1]

[25]   Kettler A, Drumm J, Heuer F, *et al.* Can a modified interspinous spacer prevent instability in axial rotation and lateral bending? A biomechanical *in vitro* study resulting in a new idea. Clin Biomech (Bristol, Avon) 2008; 23(2): 242-7.
[http://dx.doi.org/10.1016/j.clinbiomech.2007.09.004] [PMID: 17981380]

[26]   Chen HC, Wu JL, Huang SC, *et al.* Biomechanical evaluation of a novel pedicle screw-based interspinous spacer: A finite element analysis. Med Eng Phys 2017; 46: 27-32.
[http://dx.doi.org/10.1016/j.medengphy.2017.05.004] [PMID: 28622909]

[27]   Wang JC, Spenciner D, Robinson JC. SPIRE spinous process stabilization plate: biomechanical evaluation of a novel technology. J Neurosurg Spine 2006; 4(2): 160-4.
[http://dx.doi.org/10.3171/spi.2006.4.2.160] [PMID: 16506484]

[28]   Karahalios DG, Kaibara T, Porter RW, *et al.* Biomechanics of a lumbar interspinous anchor with anterior lumbar interbody fusion. J Neurosurg Spine 2010; 12(4): 372-80.
[http://dx.doi.org/10.3171/2009.10.SPINE09305] [PMID: 20367372]

[29]   Kaibara T, Karahalios DG, Porter RW, *et al.* Biomechanics of a lumbar interspinous anchor with transforaminal lumbar interbody fixation. World Neurosurg 2010; 73(5): 572-7.
[http://dx.doi.org/10.1016/j.wneu.2010.02.025] [PMID: 20920945]

[30]   Techy F, Mageswaran P, Colbrunn RW, Bonner TF, McLain RF. Properties of an interspinous fixation device (ISD) in lumbar fusion constructs: a biomechanical study. Spine J 2013; 13(5): 572-9.
[http://dx.doi.org/10.1016/j.spinee.2013.01.042] [PMID: 23498926]

[31]   Gonzalez-Blohm SA, Doulgeris JJ, Aghayev K, Lee WE III, Volkov A, Vrionis FD. Biomechanical analysis of an interspinous fusion device as a stand-alone and as supplemental fixation to posterior expandable interbody cages in the lumbar spine. J Neurosurg Spine 2014; 20(2): 209-19.
[http://dx.doi.org/10.3171/2013.10.SPINE13612] [PMID: 24286528]

[32]   Whang PG, Tran O, Rosner HL. Longitudinal comparative analysis of complications and subsequent interventions following stand-alone interspinous spacers, open decompression, or fusion for lumbar stenosis. Adv Ther 2023; 40(8): 3512-24.
[http://dx.doi.org/10.1007/s12325-023-02562-6] [PMID: 37289411]

[33]   Kumar N, Thomas AC, Rajoo MS, *et al.* Evaluating 5-year outcomes of interlaminar devices as an adjunct to decompression for symptomatic lumbar spinal stenosis. Eur Spine J 2023; 32(4): 1367-74.
[http://dx.doi.org/10.1007/s00586-023-07610-x] [PMID: 36840820]

[34]   Lewandrowski KU, Abraham I, Ramírez León JF, *et al.* A differential clinical benefit examination of full lumbar endoscopy *vs* interspinous process spacers in the treatment of spinal stenosis: an effect size meta-analysis of clinical outcomes. Int J Spine Surg 2022; 16(1): 102-23.
[http://dx.doi.org/10.14444/8200] [PMID: 35177530]

[35]   Shen H, Fogel GR, Zhu J, Liao Z, Liu W. Biomechanical analysis of lumbar fusion with proximal interspinous process device implantation. Int J Numer Methods Biomed Eng 2021; 37(8): e3498.
[http://dx.doi.org/10.1002/cnm.3498] [PMID: 33998776]

[36]   Fan W, Guo LX. Biomechanical investigation of lumbar interbody fusion supplemented with topping-off instrumentation using different dynamic stabilization devices. Spine 2021; 46(24): E1311-9.
[http://dx.doi.org/10.1097/BRS.0000000000004095] [PMID: 33958539]

[37]   Fan W, Zhang C, Zhang DX, Guo LX, Zhang M. Biomechanical analysis of lumbar nonfusion dynamic stabilization using a pedicle screw-based dynamic stabilizer or an interspinous process spacer. Int J Numer Methods Biomed Eng 2022; 38(11): e3645.
[http://dx.doi.org/10.1002/cnm.3645] [PMID: 36054421]

[38]   Fan W, Guo LX. Biomechanical investigation of topping-off technique using an interspinous process device following lumbar interbody fusion under vibration loading. Med Biol Eng Comput 2021; 59(11-12): 2449-58.
[http://dx.doi.org/10.1007/s11517-021-02458-z] [PMID: 34671891]

[39]   Lo HJ, Chen HM, Kuo YJ, Yang SW. Effect of different designs of interspinous process devices on the instrumented and adjacent levels after double-level lumbar decompression surgery: A finite element analysis. PLoS One 2020; 15(12): e0244571.
[http://dx.doi.org/10.1371/journal.pone.0244571] [PMID: 33378405]

[40]   Parchi PD, Evangelisti G, Vertuccio A, *et al.* Biomechanics of interspinous devices. BioMed Res Int 2014; 2014: 1-7.
[http://dx.doi.org/10.1155/2014/839325] [PMID: 25114923]

[41]   Schizas C, Pralong E, Tzioupis C, Kulik G. Interspinous distraction in lumbar spinal stenosis: a neurophysiological perspective. Spine 2013; 38(24): 2113-7.
[http://dx.doi.org/10.1097/01.brs.0000435031.96058.f6] [PMID: 24026157]

[42]   Marcia S, Hirsch JA, Bellini M, Manfré L, Masala S, Zini C. Percutaneous removal and replacement of a novel percutaneous interspinous device. Neuroradiol J 2023; 19714009231212366.
[PMID: 37921595]

[43]   Aggarwal N, Chow R. Real world adverse events of interspinous spacers using manufacturer and user facility device experience data. Anesth Pain Med 2021; 16(2): 177-83.
[http://dx.doi.org/10.17085/apm.20093]

[44]   Florence TJ, Say I, Patel KS, *et al.* Neurosurgical management of interspinous device complications: a case series. Front Surg 2022; 9: 841134.
[http://dx.doi.org/10.3389/fsurg.2022.841134] [PMID: 35372480]

[45]   Gazzeri R, Galarza M, Neroni M, *et al.* Failure rates and complications of interspinous process decompression devices: a European multicenter study. Neurosurg Focus 2015; 39(4): E14.
[http://dx.doi.org/10.3171/2015.7.FOCUS15244] [PMID: 26424338]

[46]   Barbagallo GMV, Olindo G, Corbino L, Albanese V. Analysis of complications in patients treated with the X-stop interspinous process decompression system: proposal for a novel anatomic scoring system for patient selection and review of the literature. Neurosurgery 2009; 65(1): 111-20.
[http://dx.doi.org/10.1227/01.NEU.0000346254.07116.31] [PMID: 19574832]

[47]   Pintauro M, Duffy A, Vahedi P, Rymarczuk G, Heller J. Interspinous implants: are the new implants better than the last generation? A review. Curr Rev Musculoskelet Med 2017; 10(2): 189-98.
[http://dx.doi.org/10.1007/s12178-017-9401-z] [PMID: 28332140]

CHAPTER 7

Biomechanical Basis of Spinal Stability and Instability Scores

Clayton Rosinski[1,*], **Asad Lak**[1], **Mani Sandhu**[1] and **Patrick W. Hitchon**[1]

[1] *University of Iowa Hospitals and Clinics, Department of Neurosurgery, Iowa City, Iowa, Unites States*

Abstract: It is critical for any doctor dealing with spinal trauma cases to be able to reliably and quickly determine the stability of traumatic injuries throughout the sub-axial spine. Ultimately, the stability of the spine is dependent on numerous, complex biomechanical relationships between bone, ligament, disc, and muscle. There have been many attempts at classifying different traumatic injuries in the spine based on mechanism, morphology, and a combination of the two, which are presented for review along with two commonly used systems in modern practice.

Keywords: Posttraumatic instability, Vertebral fracture.

INTRODUCTION

Evaluating traumatic injuries in the thoracic and lumbar spine is a large part of neurosurgical practice. To do this properly, an understanding of the biomechanics of the thoracolumbar spine is needed. The end goal of evaluating a patient with traumatic thoracolumbar injuries is to determine if said injuries result in mechanical instability of the spine, as these patients may require surgical fixation. Throughout the years, our understanding of the biomechanics of the thoracolumbar spine has been advanced through clinical observations, cadaveric studies, and computerized models of the spine. This chapter will briefly present the anatomy responsible for spinal stability and the evolution of different thoracolumbar trauma classification systems that have been developed to determine if a fracture results in spinal instability.

BIOMECHANICAL ROLE OF THORACOLUMBAR SPINAL ANATOMY

Stability of the spine refers to the ability of the spine to maintain posture, function, and neurological integrity of the contained spinal cord and cauda equina.

---
* **Corresponding author Clayton Rosinski:** University of Iowa Hospitals and Clinics, Department of Neurosurgery, Iowa City, Iowa, Unites States; E-mail: clayton-rosinski@uiowa.edu

Javier Melchor Duart Clemente (Ed.)

The mechanical stability and properties of the thoracolumbar spine are the result of a complex interplay of skeleton, ligaments, and muscles. In its entirety, the spine provides dynamic stability, which confers strength for upright position, and protection of neural elements, while allowing a finite amount of movement in all 3 planes: axial rotation, flexion and extension, and lateral bending [1].

The bony elements of the spine include the vertebral body, neural arch, spinous process, and facet processes. Anteriorly, the vertebral body is a large cylinder that provides much of the axial strength of the spine, forming a large column where the axial load is eventually transmitted to the pelvis. Additionally, the posterior portion of the vertebral body forms the anterior wall of the spinal canal. The neural arch, comprised of the pedicles, facets, and lamina, forms the lateral and posterior aspects of the spinal canal, enclosing the spinal cord and nerve roots within the bone, thereby protecting these delicate structures. The spinous process extends posteriorly off the lamina in the midline, serving as an attachment point for various muscles and ligaments of the spine, but it does not add to the bony support of the spine. Each vertebra includes two superior, and two inferior articulating facets connected by the pars interarticularis. The facet processes themselves provide strength in opposing excessive movement of the spine, providing strength in flexion and extension, opposing excessive rotation, lateral bending, and translation of one vertebra on another. Iatrogenic excision of facets, or their disruption by trauma or disease results in instability, deformity, and potential neurologic deficit [2]. The facets are necessary for preventing the translation of one vertebra into another. In the adult spine, a fracture of facets is necessary for an injury to result in translation or dislocation. Based on the orientation of the facet joints, it is easy to see why dislocation occurs most easily in the cervical spine due to the most horizontally oriented joint line, whereas dislocation in the thoracic spine is rare due to nearly vertical orientation, and translation in this segment of the spine almost always requires fracture of the facets (Fig. **1**).

The pedicles are robust bony bridges that connect the bodies to the neural arch. Congenital absence of pedicles or disruption through trauma or tumor impairs stability and alignment. In addition, pedicles are important anchors for spinal instrumentation when stability has been disrupted by trauma, tumor, or infection.

Stability of the thoracic spine is further enhanced by the rib cage which has been demonstrated in numerous cadaveric as well as computerized models. The intact rib cage further stiffens the thoracic spine, reducing motion in all planes compared to the mobile cervical and lumbar spines. It would take removal of several ribs or disarticulation of the sternum to destabilize the thoracic spine [4 - 6].

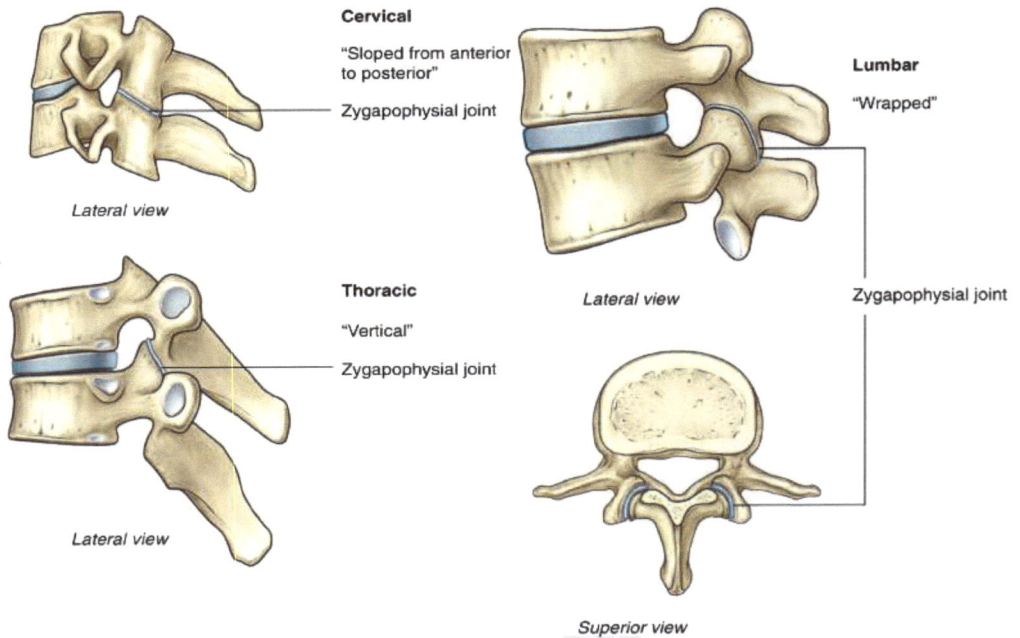

Fig. (1). Diagram comparing anatomy and orientation of cervical (least vertically oriented), thoracic (most vertically oriented), and lumbar (vertical and angled in the axial plane) facet joints. Courtesy of Drake RL, Vogl W, Mitchell AWM, Gray H. Gray's anatomy for students. Fourth edition [3].

The vertebral bodies of adjacent vertebrae are separated by and connected to each other *via* an intervertebral disc. The disc is composed of two parts, the fibrous, exterior limiting structure called the *annulus fibrosus* which contains the inner gel-like material termed *nucleus pulposus*. The *annulus fibrosus* is made of collagenous fibers arranged in laminated bands, which are oriented 90 degrees to the adjacent band. At the bony interface, the *annulus* attaches to the cartilaginous end plate of the vertebral body as well as the cortical surface of the body. The *annulus* confers resistance to rotation, tensile, and shear stresses, which helps prevent excessive movement in any plane or rotation between two adjacent vertebral bodies. The *nucleus pulposus* is made of mucopolysaccharides, mucoprotein, and water forming a gel that forms a viscoelastic material whose mechanical properties change with changing rates at an applied load. The slower a load is applied, the greater the *nucleus pulposus* can deform, and *vice versa*, which helps provide motion to the spine with purposeful movement but can fail under severe traumatic impacts. Additionally, in the axial load, the nucleus acts to absorb shock, cushioning the spine.

Much of the stability of the spine is due to the seven elastin and collagen-composed ligaments which connect various bony structures of the spine between adjacent vertebra and sometimes across numerous spinal segments (Fig. **2**). Anteriorly to the entirety of the spinal column is the anterior longitudinal ligament (ALL); in totality, the ALL functions to prevent hyperextension of the spine. In parallel to the ALL, the posterior longitudinal ligament (PLL) is bound to the posterior portion of the vertebral column within the spinal canal, attaching to the posterior aspects of the vertebral body and interwoven with the posterior *annulus fibrosus*; the PLL helps resist hyperflexion. The *ligamentum flavum* is a discontinuous ligament that attaches adjacent lamina on their anterior surface within the spinal canal. Laterally, the *ligamenta flava* are intertwined with the facet capsule. The *ligamentum flavum* does not limit flexion but becomes taut when returning to a neutral position in extension. The facet capsule forms between the articulating facet processes of the adjacent vertebra forming the limits of the facet joint, which is critical to the strength in resisting excessive motion provided by this joint. Posteriorly, the interspinous ligament connects adjacent spinous processes extending from the base to the tip of each spinous process. The supraspinous ligament is a continuous ligament extending from the tip of the C7 spinous process down throughout the spine attaching to the tip of each spinous process. Together, the interspinous or infraspinous, and supraspinous ligaments provide considerable resistance to hyperflexion, as they act on a long moment of the posterior neural arch [7].

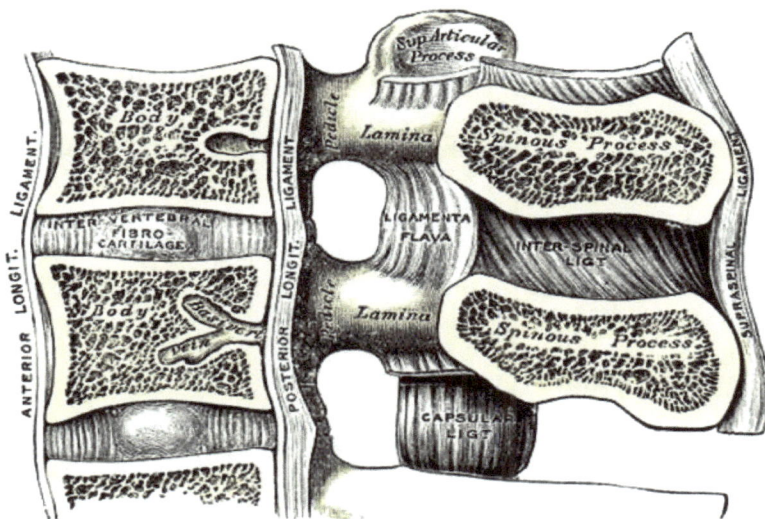

Fig. (2). Diagram of the ligamentous components of the functional spine unit. Original diagram from Gray's anatomy, now out of copyright. This diagram has been reproduced from Gray's Anatomy 20th US edition which has now lapsed into the public domain (https://commons.wikimedia.org/wiki/File:Gray301.png).

The above-described structures (bony elements, intervertebral disc, facet joint, and ligaments) of a pair of adjacent vertebrae form the functional spinal unit. The functional unit of the spine is what confers the ability of the spine to allow for some motion while maintaining mechanical stability. The components of the functional spine unit are not the only structures that influence the motion and stability of the spine, as both the spinal musculature and rib cage add stability to the spine. In the thoracic spine, the anterior thoracic cage provides considerable bending stiffness in flexion and even more so in extension. Additionally, it adds considerable resistance to buckling of the spine under axial load. There are numerous muscles that attach to the spine, which maintain the load balanced along the spine through complex relationships. The musculature helps offload the forces impaired on the spine, and also plays an important role in preventing progressive deformity of the spine [1].

HISTORICAL EVOLUTION OF THORACOLUMBAR TRAUMA CLASSIFICATION SYSTEMS

Defining Instability

The goal of each classification system or schema that had been devised for characterizing thoracolumbar injuries was to determine if such injuries compromised the stability of the spine. With each new report of thoracolumbar trauma came a slight variation in the definition of spinal stability. White and Panjabi described instability as "the ability of the spine under physiologic loads to limit patterns of displacement so as not to damage or irritate the spinal cord or nerve roots and, in addition, to prevent incapacitating deformity or pain due to structural changes" [8]. Therefore, an unstable spine does not have the structural strength to resist an abnormal amount of movement under the loads experienced in everyday life to prevent abnormal amounts of movement of vertebral bodies, which could lead to the compression of neural elements. It is important to note that instability allows for progressive changes, meaning that there may not be neurologic compromise at the time of the injury, but it could develop in the future if stability is not restored.

Holdsworth's Two-Column Spine Model

In 1962, Sir Frank Holdsworth published the idea of a two-column spinal model in his landmark paper where he described different fractures, dislocations, and fracture-dislocations of the spine based on his observations from managing thousands of patients with traumatic spine injuries at the Sheffield Spinal Injuries Centre [9]. Holdsworth described the posterior ligamentous complex (PLC) as the supraspinous and interspinous ligaments, facet joint capsules, and *ligamentum flava*. He surmised that the stability of the spine after an injury is dependent on the integrity of the PLC, the fibers of which rarely rupture from a purely longitudinal force-experienced during pure flexion-, but readily tear with twisting or rotation. With this in mind, he proposed the two-column spine model, in which the spine only became destabilized if there was injury to both the anterior column (vertebral body, disc, ALL, and PLL) and posterior column (neural arch, PLC). He then went on to characterize five types of spine injuries based on the mechanism of injury and whether they were stable or not. These include pure flexion, flexion rotation, extension, vertebral compression, and shearing. Pure flexion, extension, and vertebral compression injuries were all deemed stable. The two fractures which, by the two-column system are determined unstable are flexion rotation and shearing.

Denis's Three-Column Spine Model

In 1983, Francis Denis published a paper on Holdsworth's two-column model with the addition of a third column, which emphasized the importance of the posterior disc *annulus* [10]. This model was devised from a retrospective study of 412 trauma cases as well as the incorporation of numerous studies, which showed that pure disruption of the PLC alone did not result in instability, but that disruption of the PLL and posterior *annulus* was required for instability [11 - 15]. Denis described the middle column of the spine as the posterior vertebral body wall, PLL, and posterior *annulus*. This leaves the anterior column as the ALL and anterior 2/3 of the vertebral body, and the posterior column being the posterior arch and PLC (Fig. 3). Denis then characterized thoracolumbar trauma into four different patterns.

A. Compression fractures (Fig. 4) are characterized by anterior column failure under compression. This occurs during compression and flexion where the middle column acts as a hinge as it remains intact. Extreme cases occur where there is partial tension failure of the PLC. These fractures can occur both anteriorly and laterally depending on the direction of flexion. These are considered stable but can develop progressive deformity.

B. Burst fractures (Fig. 5) result in failure of the anterior and middle columns under an axial load. The anterior and posterior vertebral body cortex both fractures resulting in a loss of both anterior and posterior body height loss. There is also an increase in the interpedicular distance and possible greenstick fracture of the anterior cortex of the lamina. In the lumbar spine, there is rarely any kyphotic deformity, which can be seen at the thoracolumbar junction as an axial load in this area often results in flexion. Mechanically stable, but can result in both immediate or progressive neurologic deficit upon ambulation, as the increased axial load results in further retropulsion of the burst fragments.

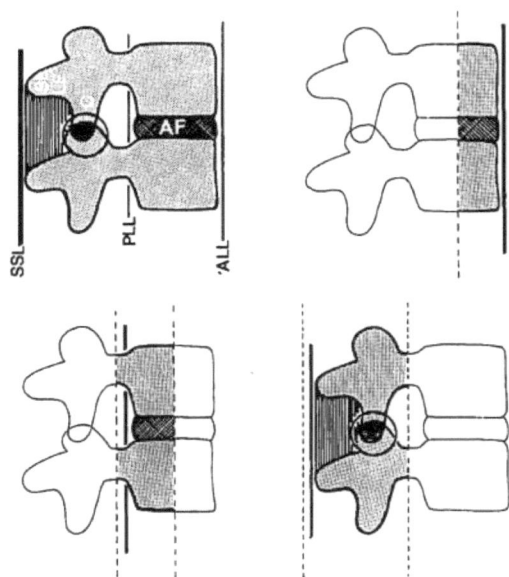

Fig. (3). Three spinal columns were devised by Denis. The anterior column (top right) is composed of ALL, anterior annulus, and anterior vertebral body. The middle column (bottom left) is composed of PLL, posterior annulus, and posterior vertebral body. The posterior column (bottom right) is comprised of SSL, ISL, posterior arch, facet capsule, and *ligamentum flavum*.

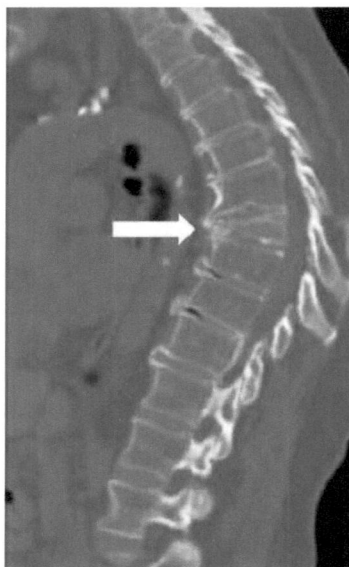

Fig. (4). Thoracic compression fracture (arrow) in a woman in her 60s with a history of chronic obstructive pulmonary disease on chronic steroids. She denies any specific accident or injury. Clinically there is pain without neurological deficit. Radiologically there is kyphosis, loss in height, but no dislocation. Treatment is bracing and analgesic, being kyphoplasty an option in case intractable pain develops.

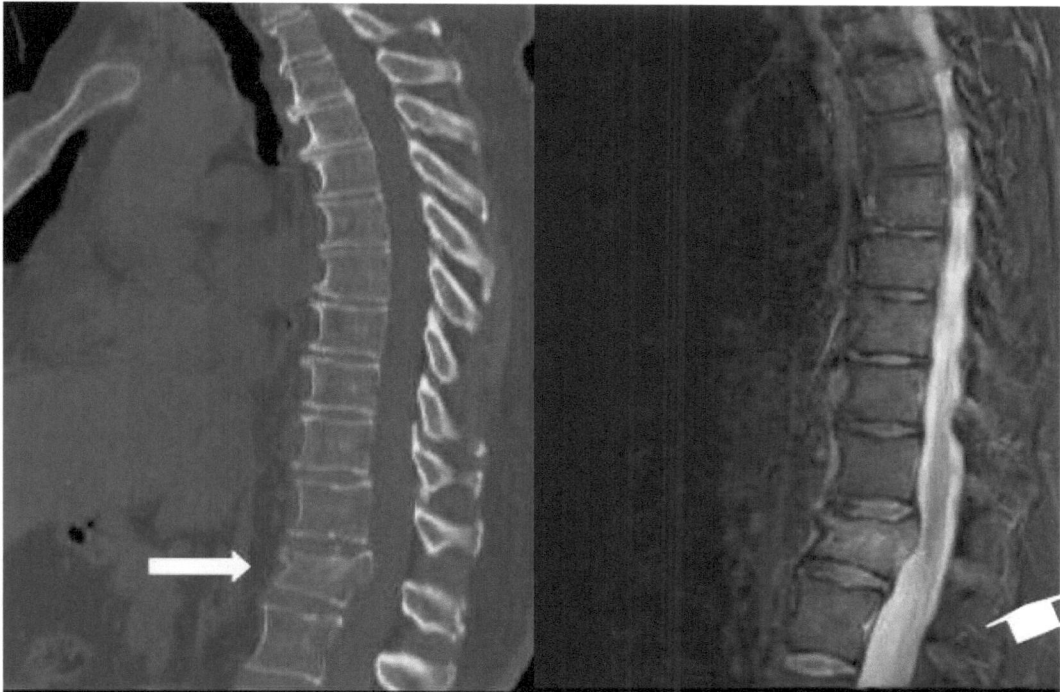

Fig. (5). A female in her 50s was admitted after a fall down 12-14 stairs while intoxicated. She is neurologically intact, just with pain. CT (left) and MRI (right) display a burst fracture of T12 with retropulsion of bone (arrow, left image), without disruption of the PLC (lack of hyper intensity noted by arrow, right image). She was placed in a back brace, with gradual resolution of her pain. She was off the narcotic pain medications after 10 days.

C. Seatbelt-type injuries (Fig. **6**) are primarily flexion distraction injuries but also include Chance fractures. In these fractures, there is flexion ± distraction where the spine hinges over the anterior column resulting in disruption of the medial and posterior columns due to tension forces generated by extreme flexion. There can be failure of the anterior column as well, but it must be able to act as a hinge. This results in increased posterior body height due to a horizontal fracture of the posterior cortex, posterior disc space, or pedicles. If this occurs within a single level where all ligaments from the PLL and posteriorly are disrupted, it is referred to as a Chance fracture, which was first described by GQ Chance, a radiologist, in 1948 [16]. These injuries often involve two adjacent levels, which are differentiated by whether the posterior body cortex or posterior *annulus* is disrupted. These often do not have immediate mechanical instability but are at very high risk for progressive deformity and instability.

D. Fracture dislocation results in failure of all three columns resulting in subluxation or dislocation of the spine (Fig. **7**). Three subclassifications of these fractures were characterized based on the mechanism of injury. Flexion-rotation injuries resulted in complete rupture of the middle and posterior columns due to tension and rotational forces, while the anterior column failed due to compression and rotation. There is often stripping of the ALL off the anterior body due to rotation, which is the cause of three-column failure. The middle column fails either due to disruption of the posterior disc or a fracture through the posterior body (slice fracture). The second subtype is a shear-type fracture dislocation, where all three columns are disrupted including the ALL due to force-directed directly onto the spine typically in the posteroanterior direction. Ultimately, there is complete shearing of the superior portion of the spine from the inferior portion. Lastly, the flexion-distraction subtype was characterized, which is like the seatbelt injury but accompanied by complete disc disruption resulting in anterior column failure allowing subluxation or dislocation. These injuries result in both mechanical and neurologic instability.

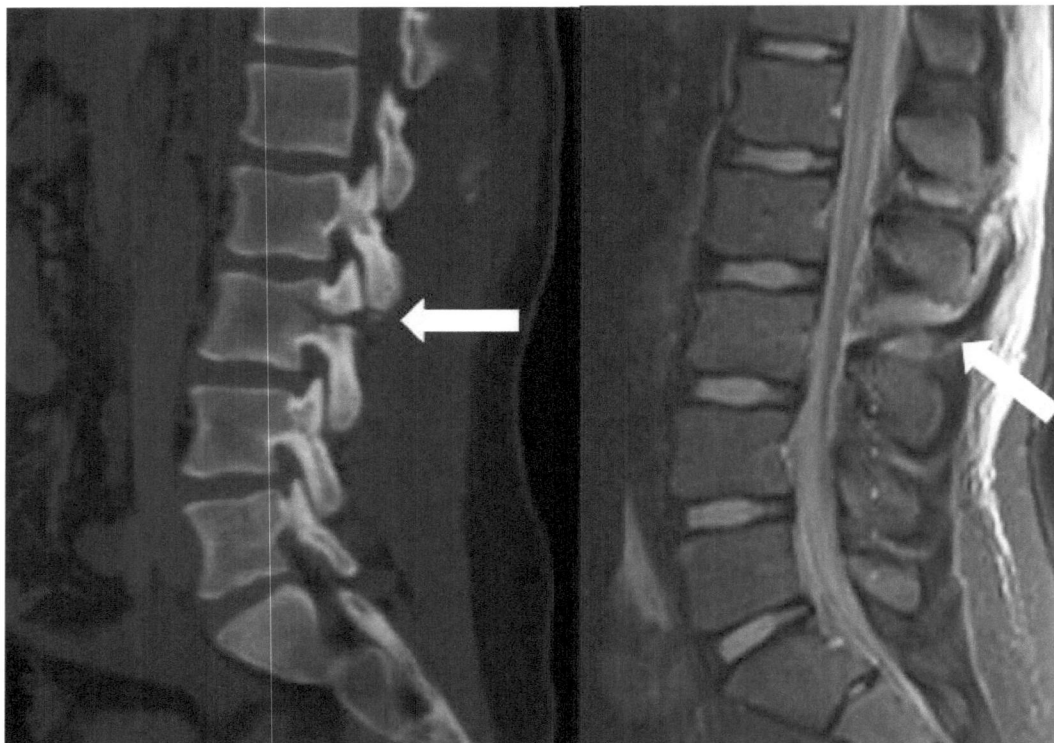

Fig. (6). An adolescent male was involved in a motor vehicle accident. He complained of back pain but had no neurological deficit. CT imaging (left) revealed a flexion-distraction fracture of L3 extending through the body and pedicles (arrow). Stir sequence MRI (right) revealed the ligamentous injury to the posterior ligamentous complex (hyperintensity indicated by the arrow). Surgery consisted of minimally invasive pedicle screw fixation to restore the posterior tension band.

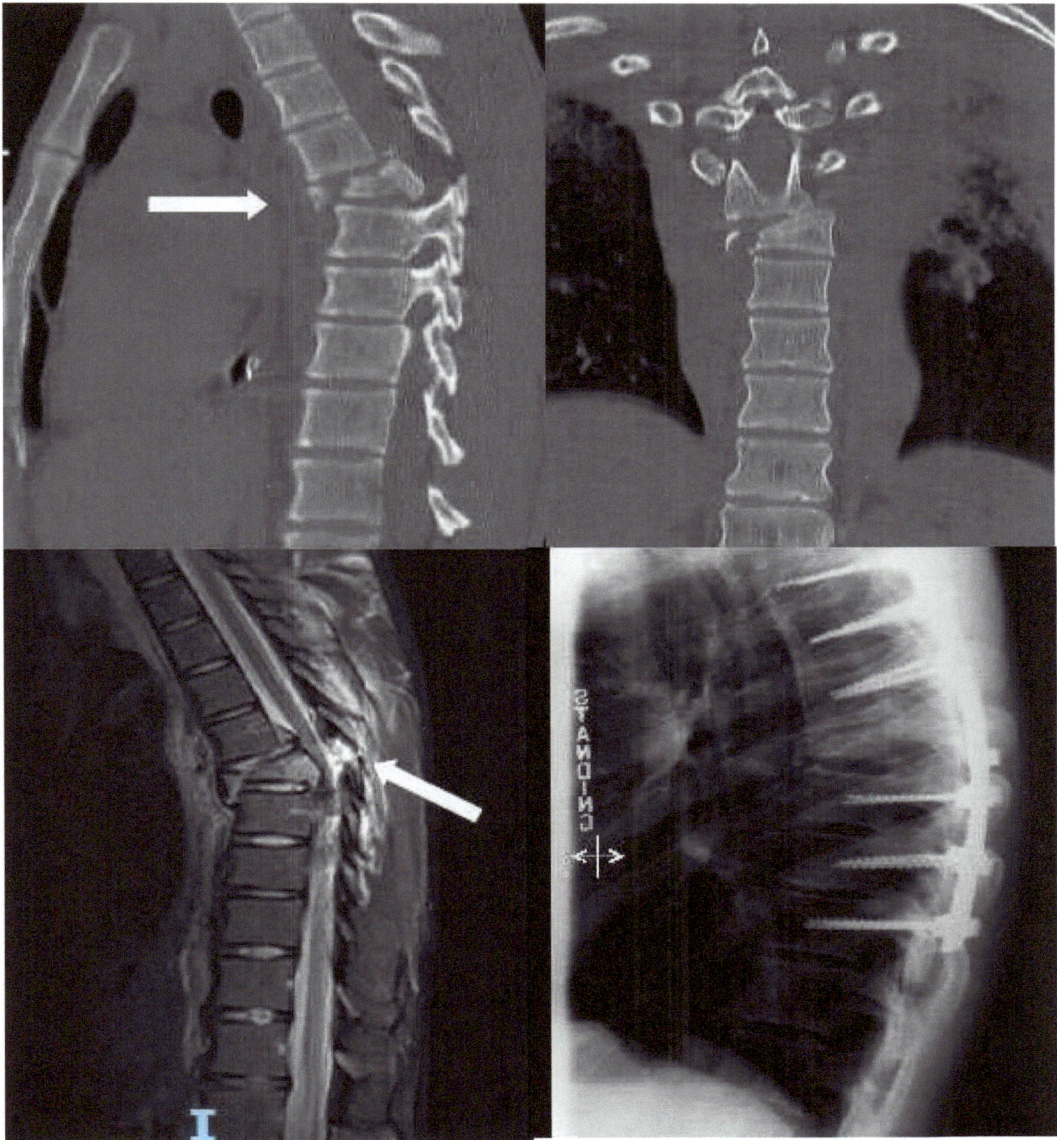

Fig. (7). A young adult male was the unrestrained driver in a vehicle traveling at highway speeds and ejected 40 feet. He was initially unresponsive but was able to move all 4 extremities. CT (top left) shows fracture dislocation of T6 on T7 (arrow). Coronal CT (top right) shows lateral displacement of T6 on T7. STIR MRI (bottom left) shows ligamentous disruption of discs and PLC (arrow). He was treated with posterior instrumentation (bottom right). On follow-up 18 months later he was neurologically intact, and hardware was removed.

Panjabi and White three column instability score

An algorithm that combines the above concepts of stable and unstable spinal fractures was put forth by Panjabi and White in 1978, and in several publications since then. This algorithm facilitates, then and now, patient management and has withstood the erosion of time.

Thoracolumbar Injury Classification and Severity Score (TLICS)

In 2005, a group led by Alexander Vaccaro published a paper where a new classification system for thoracolumbar traumatic injuries was developed through a review of previous literature followed by the creation of a scale with a panel of 40 spine surgeons from trauma centers around the world [17]. The system was then validated in subsequent surveys. What was unique about the TLICS system, was that it not only classified these injuries but provided a management recommendation based on the scoring system. The other major strength of the scale was its simplicity, lending itself to great ease of use in the clinical setting. The scale is comprised of three main components: fracture pattern, PLC integrity, and neurologic function.

The pattern of fracture is based on imaging findings and is important regarding the immediate stability of an injury. Compression fractures are failures of the vertebral body under axial load, ranging from simple compression fractures to burst fractures, which are assigned one additional point compared to compression/wedge fractures. Translational or rotation fractures often occur from torsional and shear forces; they are much more unstable than compression fractures, as the ability to resist rotation has been lost either due to facet disruption *via* fracture or dislocation. Lastly, and most unstable, is the distraction injury morphology, where two parts of the spinal column have been disrupted circumferentially. This requires either disruption of both anterior and posterior ligament, anterior and posterior bony element fractures, or a combination of both. By default, these injuries are unstable.

The integrity of the PLC (supraspinous ligament, interspinous ligament, *ligamentum flavum*, and facet capsules) is important in determining management, as it prevents excessive flexion, rotation, translation, and distraction. Additionally, the PLC has a poor ability to heal, further increasing the importance of its integrity. The integrity of the PLC is indicative that an injury will have long-term stability, as if it is disrupted the risk of progressive deformity is much greater. This is assessed primarily through imaging, where disruption can be seen directly with MRI, or indirectly *via* splaying of the spinous processes, facet diastasis, perching or subluxation, and vertebral body translation or rotation. This may not always be clear, which is why indeterminate can be assigned.

Lastly, neurologic function is included in the scale. This inclusion was novel, as it was the first time the patient's exam was taken into consideration for thoracolumbar traumatic injury classification. Neurologic status is seen as an indicator of the severity of the injury and can be the reason alone to pursue surgical intervention. Patients are examined and interviewed to determine whether they are intact, have a nerve root injury, complete spinal cord injury, and most significantly, either an incomplete cord injury or cauda equina syndrome. These factors are each assessed and then scored per the scale (Table **1**). Based on the cumulative opinion of the 40 surgeons involved in developing the scale, injuries scored 3 or less should be managed nonoperative, 5 or more with surgery, and 4 can be handled conservatively or surgically. The authors went beyond just recommending the type of management but even provided recommendations for a surgical approach based on the neurologic status of the patient and the integrity of the PLC (Tables **2** and **3**). However, each surgical intervention will be dictated by a patient's specific injury pattern and other patient-specific factors.

Table 1. TLICS scoring criteria and management recommendation.

Injury Morphology	Points	
Compression	1	
Burst	2	
Translational/rotational	3	
Distraction	4	
Integrity of the Posterior Ligamentous Complex		
Intact		0
Suspected/indeterminate		2
Injured (disrupted in tension, rotation, or translation)		3
Neurologic Status Involvement Qualifiers		
Intact	-	0
Nerve Root	-	2
Cord, conus medullaris	Complete	2
-	Incomplete	3
Cauda equina	-	3
Management Recommendation of Score		
Score	Management	
0-3	Conservative (nonsurgical management)	
4	Surgeon's preference	
5-10	Surgical	

Table 2. Checklist for the diagnosis of clinical instability of the thoracic spine.

Element	Point Value
Anterior elements destroyed	2
Posterior elements destroyed	2
Disruption of costovertebral articulation	1
Sagittal displacement >2.5mm	2
Sagittal plane angulation >5°	2
Spinal cord or cauda equina damage	2
Dangerous loading anticipated	1
A total score ≥ 5 indicates clinical instability.	

Table 3. Checklist for the diagnosis of clinical instability of the lumbar spine.

Element	point Value
Anterior elements destroyed	2
Posterior elements destroyed	2
Cauda equina damage	3
Relative flexion sagittal plane translation >8% or extension sagittal plane translation >9%	2
Relative flexion sagittal plane rotation >9%	2
A total score ≥ 5 indicates clinical instability.	

HISTORICAL EVOLUTION OF CERVICAL TRAUMA CLASSIFICATION SYSTEMS

Introduction

The spinal column serves as the body's center of gravity, allowing the head to be rested on top of the pelvis. The spinal column achieves this function *via* an interplay between vertebrae, ligaments, and joints, each of which permits variable degrees of movement. The vertebral body in conjunction with the intervertebral disc disseminates the axial load. In contrast, the posterior ligamentous complex in collaboration with facet joints acts as a tension band and resists excessive flexion, extension, or rotation. Any interruption of this physiological relationship between various segments of the spinal column will lead to instability. Hence, an understanding of spinal biomechanics is critical in understanding spinal trauma and its implications.

The sub-axial cervical spine, which comprises C3-C7, is frequently affected by trauma. Sub-axial cervical spine trauma accounts for the majority of cervical spine trauma and accounts for 65% of fractures and 75% of dislocations [18].

Holdsworth classification

A basic understanding of the biomechanics of the spinal column and the implications of traumatic cervical fractures was first provided by Sir Frank Holdsworth [9]. He divided the sub-axial cervical spine into two columns: the anterior column comprising the vertebral body, intervertebral disc, and anterior and posterior longitudinal ligaments, and the posterior column comprising the articular process, facet capsule, pedicle, lamina, and posterior ligamentous complex comprising *ligamentum flavum,* interspinous and supraspinous ligaments. Based on his observations, he stated that posterior ligamentous complex and facet joints are the most important determinants for the pattern of injury. Based on his observations, he described six patterns of fractures: compression, burst, extension, dislocation, rotational fracture dislocation, and shear fracture. The biomechanical rationale for his classification system was that each type of fracture resulted from a distinct force, differing in intensity and direction of action. He further went on and recommended surgical treatment for only unstable fractures, which included dislocation, rotational fracture dislocation, and shear fractures.

Allen's classification

In 1982, Allen *et al.* built on the work done by Holdsworth and proposed his classification system [19]. The underlying biomechanical rationale was that in addition to the direction of force, the posture of the cervical spine at the time of impact is also important. They classified cervical spine trauma under the following broad categories: **1**. Compressive flexion **2**. Vertical compression **3**. Distractive Flexion **4**. Compressive Extension **5**. Distractive Extension **6**. Lateral Flexion. Within these broad categories, they further described further subtypes based on the severity of injury. This system, even though including more mechanistic detail about sub-axial cervical spine fracture than Holdsworth, is however more complicated, has poor reliability, and was never employed in clinical practice.

Harris classification

Based on further clinical, radiographic, and cadaveric evidence, another classification system was proposed by Harris *et al.* to obtain a practical classification method for cervical spine trauma [20]. The authors postulated that a cervical spine classification system needs to be simple, replicable, and able to describe the mechanism for underlying injury. They built on the spinal column theory proposed by Holdsworth and Dennis *et al.* and stated that a particular injury results from one predominant vector force or a combination of forces acting along a particular axis of the body *e.g.*, horizontal, sagittal, or coronal. They also postulated that several different types of injuries can be produced by the same force and that the magnitude of injury is directly proportional to the magnitude of force. The classification proposed ultimately categorized different types of fractures based on the predominant force that caused such an injury (Table **4**).

Table 4. Harris cervical fracture classification.

Predominant Force	INJURY SUBTYPE
Flexion	-
-	Hyperflexion sprain
-	Bilateral facet dislocation
-	Compression fracture
-	Clay-shoveler fracture
-	Flexion teardrop fracture
Flexion rotation	-
Extension	-
Vertical compression	-
-	Jefferson fracture of the atlas
-	Burst fracture
Hyperextension	-
-	Hyperextension dislocation
-	Avulsion fracture of atlas anterior arch
-	Extension teardrop fracture of axis
-	Fracture of posterior atlas arch
-	-
-	Laminar fracture
-	Traumatic spondylolisthesis (Hangman's)
-	Hyperextension fracture-dislocation
Lateral flexion	-
Diverse/poorly understood.	-
-	Atlanto-occipital dissociation
-	Odontoid fracture

Cervical Spine Injury Severity Score (CSISS)

While previous classification systems focused on biomechanical principles and provided a morphological classification system, there was still a need for a clinically useful system that could assess prognosis and guide treatment strategy. This was sensed by Anderson *et al.* and a new classification system was proposed [21]. The Spinal Trauma Study Group (STSG) devised its own system which focused on the stability of the spinal column in addition to the mechanism of injury and morphology of fracture. They also stated that the patient's neurological function should be given importance while deciding treatment strategy, however, neurological status was not formally included in the classification system. Moreover, the Spine Trauma Study Group proposed that instability should be graded on a continuum rather than as a binary variable.

This system subdivides the sub-axial cervical spine into four columns; the anterior column that comprises the vertebral body, intervertebral disc, uncinate process, anterior longitudinal ligament, and posterior longitudinal ligament; the posterior column comprises bilateral lamina, spinous process, *ligamentum flavum* and posterior longitudinal complex; right and left lateral columns comprising the pedicle, lateral mass, superior and inferior articular process, facet capsule and transverse process. Assessment of stability was based on the severity of bony and ligamentous disruption, which was subsequently assessed based on the degree of skeletal displacement or osseous dissociation. Each column was given a score from 0-5 with 0 indicating no injury and 5 indicating the worst possible injury. The total possible score was 20 on this scale with the assumption that multi-column injuries will result in higher scores.

One of the advantages of this system is the higher degree of intra-observer and inter-observer reliability. The authors noticed an association between score and clinical decision-making as a cumulative score > 7 resulted in surgery in 100% of cases. Moreover, an association was observed between neurological status and overall score as a score >7 was associated with neurological deficit in 80% of cases. However, this system has not been validated and is too cumbersome for clinical practice.

Sub-axial Cervical Spine Injury Classification System (SLICS) scale

The Spinal Trauma Study group comprising 50 surgeons from 12 countries around the world reviewed the available literature on sub-axial cervical spine trauma. The group noted that the current classification systems [22] are not only cumbersome and impractical to use in clinical practice, but they also rely on plain radiographs and ignore the role of ligamentous injury and the patient's neurological status. To address this issue, they devised a novel classification system that not only provides information about the pattern and severity of injury but also guides treatment decision-making and the patient's prognosis [23]. It was also noted that parameters found to be important in treatment decision-making for thoracolumbar trauma (TLICS) were also useful predictors of outcome in sub-axial cervical spine trauma [17].

Based on the literature review and experience of STSG committee members, several different injury characteristics noted to be important in sub-axial cervical spine trauma were identified. Weighted scores were provided for fracture pattern, disco-ligamentous complex injury, and the patient's neurological status (Table **5**). The total score was calculated by summing individual scores. The new classification system was then applied to 11 different cases of sub-axial trauma. The intra-observer and inter-observer reliability of the system was calculated based on the assessment of surgeons. Moreover, the validity of the classification system was assessed by experts in the field of cervical spine trauma by comparing SLIC scores with an independent assessment of whether the case is surgical or not. The newer classification system had moderate intra-rater and inter-rater reliability, which compared favorably with older classification systems. The SLIC scale demonstrated a higher construct validity as raters agreed with treatment recommendations in 93.3% of cases. Based on the SLIC scale, injuries with a score of> 5 need surgical intervention (Fig. **8**), and injuries with a score <3 of should be managed non-operatively. Cases with an SLIC score of 4 were attributed treatment based on the surgeon's decision-making.

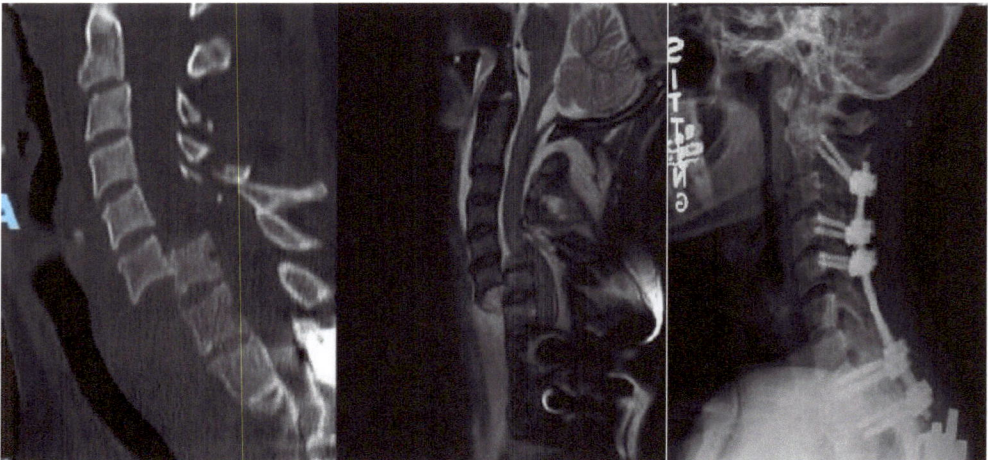

Fig. (8). The adult female involved in a motorcycle accident at highway speed. Presents with ASIA A neurological status with additional head injuries. The patient has spinal surgery for correction of scoliosis as a juvenile. CT (top left) shows fracture dislocation with spondylosis of C6 on C7. STIR MRI (top right) 3-column ligamentous injury with cord distortion and contusion. She required traction, reduction, and instrumentation (bottom left).

Table 5. SLIC scoring criteria and management recommendation.

Injury morphology	Qualifiers	Points
Type	-	-
Compression	-	1
Burst	-	2
Distraction	-	3
Rotation/translation	-	4
Integrity of the disco-ligamentous complex (DLC)		
-		-
Intact		0
Suspected/indeterminate		1
Injured (disrupted in tension, rotation, or translation)		2
Neurologic status involvement		
-	-	-
Intact	-	0
Nerve Root	-	1
Cord injury	Complete	2
-	Incomplete	3
-	Continuous compression	+1
-	-	-
Management Recommendation of Score		
Score	Management	
0-3	Conservative (nonsurgical management)	
4	Surgeon's preference	
5-10	Surgical	

CONCLUSION

Understanding the anatomy and physiology of the human vertebrae is crucial to perceive the concept of stability, the fracture patterns and when surgical treatment is considered necessary to carry on with normal life activities.

Different classifications have evolved based primarily on biomechanical principles, though clinical neurological situation has also been incorporated; knowledge and application of these scales can help the surgeon to decide which could be the best treatment option.

REFERENCES

[1] Hitchon PW, Traynelis VC, Rengachary SS, Traynelis VT, Eds. Techniques in spinal fusion and stabilization 1995. [u.a.]

[2] Zeng Z, Zhu R, Wu Y, *et al.* Effect of graded facetectomy on lumbar biomechanics. J Healthc Eng 2017; 2017: 1-6.
[http://dx.doi.org/10.1155/2017/7981513] [PMID: 29065645]

[3] Drake RL, Vogl W, Mitchell AWM, Gray H. Gray's anatomy for students 4th ed., 2020.

[4] Watkins R IV, Watkins R III, Williams L, *et al.* Stability provided by the sternum and rib cage in the thoracic spine. Spine 2005; 30(11): 1283-6.
[http://dx.doi.org/10.1097/01.brs.0000164257.69354.bb] [PMID: 15928553]

[5] Andriacchi T, Schultz A, Belytschko T, Galante J. A model for studies of mechanical interactions between the human spine and rib cage. J Biomech 1974; 7(6): 497-507.
[http://dx.doi.org/10.1016/0021-9290(74)90084-0] [PMID: 4452675]

[6] Liebsch C, Wilke HJ. Rib presence, anterior rib cage integrity, and segmental length affect the stability of the human thoracic spine: An *in vitro* study. Front Bioeng Biotechnol 2020; 8: 46.
[http://dx.doi.org/10.3389/fbioe.2020.00046] [PMID: 32117927]

[7] Steinmetz MP, Benzel EC, Eds. Benzel's spine surgery: techniques, complication avoidance, and management 4th ed., 2017.

[8] Panjabi MM, White AA III. Basic biomechanics of the spine. Neurosurgery 1980; 7(1): 76-93.
[http://dx.doi.org/10.1227/00006123-198007000-00014] [PMID: 7413053]

[9] Holdsworth F. Fractures, dislocations, and fracture-dislocations of the spine. J Bone Joint Surg Am 1970; 52(8): 1534-51.
[http://dx.doi.org/10.2106/00004623-197052080-00002] [PMID: 5483077]

[10] Denis F. The three column spine and its significance in the classification of acute thoracolumbar spinal injuries. Spine 1983; 8(8): 817-31.
[http://dx.doi.org/10.1097/00007632-198311000-00003] [PMID: 6670016]

[11] Bedbrook GM. Stability of spinal fractures and fracture dislocations. Paraplegia 1971; 9(1): 23-32.
[PMID: 5120039]

[12] DECOULX P, RIEUNAU G. Les fractures du rachis dorso-lombaire sans troubles nerveux Fractures of the dorsolumbar spine without neurological disorders. Rev Chir Orthop Reparatrice Appar Mot. 1958 Jul-Sep;44(3-4):254-322. French.
[PMID: 13602358]

[13] Panjabi MM, White AA III, Johnson RM. Cervical spine mechanics as a function of transection of components. J Biomech 1975; 8(5): 327-36.
[http://dx.doi.org/10.1016/0021-9290(75)90085-8] [PMID: 1184604]

[14] Purcell GA, Markolf KL, Dawson eg. Twelfth thoracic-first lumbar vertebral mechanical stability of fractures after Harrington-rod instrumentation. J Bone Joint Surg Am 1981; 63(1): 71-8.
[http://dx.doi.org/10.2106/00004623-198163010-00009] [PMID: 7451528]

[15] Reuber M, Schultz A, Denis F, Spencer D. Bulging of lumbar intervertebral disks. J Biomech Eng 1982; 104(3): 187-92.
[http://dx.doi.org/10.1115/1.3138347] [PMID: 7120942]

[16] Chance GQ. Note on a type of flexion fracture of the spine. Br J Radiol 1948; 21(249): 452-3.
[http://dx.doi.org/10.1259/0007-1285-21-249-452] [PMID: 18878306]

[17] Vaccaro AR, Lehman RA Jr, Hurlbert RJ, *et al.* A new classification of thoracolumbar injuries: the importance of injury morphology, the integrity of the posterior ligamentous complex, and neurologic status. Spine 2005; 30(20): 2325-33.
[http://dx.doi.org/10.1097/01.brs.0000182986.43345.cb] [PMID: 16227897]

[18]   Watson-Jones R. The results of postural reduction of fractures of the spine. J Bone Joint Surg Am 1938; 20(3): 567-86.

[19]   Allen BL Jr, Ferguson RL, Lehmann TR, O'BRIEN RP. A mechanistic classification of closed, indirect fractures and dislocations of the lower cervical spine. Spine 1982; 7(1): 1-27.
[http://dx.doi.org/10.1097/00007632-198200710-00001] [PMID: 7071658]

[20]   Harris JH Jr, Edeiken-Monroe B, Kopaniky DR. A practical classification of acute cervical spine injuries. Orthop Clin North Am 1986; 17(1): 15-30.
[http://dx.doi.org/10.1016/S0030-5898(20)30415-6] [PMID: 3511428]

[21]   Anderson PA, Moore TA, Davis KW, *et al.* Cervical spine injury severity score. Assessment of reliability. J Bone Joint Surg Am 2007; 89(5): 1057-65.
[http://dx.doi.org/10.2106/JBJS.F.00684] [PMID: 17473144]

[22]   Kim CW, Perry A, Garfin SR. Spinal instability: the orthopedic approach. Semin Musculoskelet Radiol 2005; 9(1): 77-87.
[http://dx.doi.org/10.1055/s-2005-867098] [PMID: 15812714]

[23]   Vaccaro AR, Hulbert RJ, Patel AA, *et al.* The subaxial cervical spine injury classification system: a novel approach to recognize the importance of morphology, neurology, and integrity of the disco-ligamentous complex. Spine 2007; 32(21): 2365-74.
[http://dx.doi.org/10.1097/BRS.0b013e3181557b92] [PMID: 17906580]

SUBJECT INDEX

www.ingramcontent.com/pod-product-compliance
Lightning Source LLC
Chambersburg PA
CBHW041446210326
41599CB00004B/149